An Insider's Guide to Orthopedic Surgery

A Physical Therapist Shares the Keys to a Better Recovery

ELIZABETH KAUFMANN

With a Foreword by Jared Foran, M.D.
Director of Joint Replacement Surgery,
OrthoColorado Hospital and St. Anthony Hospital

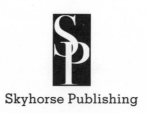

Skyhorse Publishing

Skyhorse Publishing books may be purchased in bulk at special discounts for sales promotion, corporate gifts, fund-raising, or educational purposes. Special editions can also be created to specifications. For details, contact the Special Sales Department, Skyhorse Publishing, 307 West 36th Street, 11th Floor, New York, NY 10018 or info@skyhorsepublishing.com.

Skyhorse® and Skyhorse Publishing® are registered trademarks of Skyhorse Publishing, Inc.®, a Delaware corporation.

Visit our website at www.skyhorsepublishing.com.

10 9 8 7 6 5 4 3 2 1

Library of Congress Cataloging-in-Publication Data is available on file.

Cover design by Rain Saukas
Cover photo credit: iStock

Print ISBN: 978-1-5107-2344-3
Ebook ISBN: 978-1-5107-2345-0

Printed in the United States of America

This book is intended for reference only; it is not a definitive medical manual. The information is provided to help you make decisions regarding your health and recovery, but it is not intended to replace advice and treatment from health-care providers.

Mention of specific brand name products, authorities, companies, and organizations does not imply endorsement of these by the author or publisher.

With the exception of the author's husband, names of patients and colleagues have been changed throughout.

An Insider's Guide to Orthopedic Surgery

Dedication

In memory of my mom, Elizabeth Passavant Kaufmann, whose name I share. Despite her rheumatoid arthritis diagnosis and the need for multiple joint replacements, Mom was still riding a horse at 86.

To my husband, writer Ernie Tucker, who gently critiqued this book, bolstered me throughout, and quelled my anxiety, often with comic relief. His own favorite memory of knee replacement was, without a doubt, the heated blankets.

Table of Contents

Foreword

The book you are about to read is a resource that I wish had been available for my patients a long time ago. Since the start of my career, I have been passionate about continually improving patient experiences and outcomes. It has been my observation that the simplest way to achieve this is to set realistic expectations and to empower patients for success.

Elizabeth Kaufmann, a physical therapist who has worked masterfully with my patients over the years, understands this too. Her experience treating thousands of orthopedic patients has allowed her to reflect on the elements that differentiate the average and the superstar patient. As you will learn from this book, successful surgery goes well beyond the skilled hands of the surgeon.

It is my sincere belief that there is a recipe for success after elective orthopedic surgery. What may be surprising is that I also believe that 90 percent of this recipe depends on the patient and 10 percent on the surgeon! One might wonder how this is possible. Patients often, and understandably so, spend a tremendous amount of time trying to find the right surgeon, but not enough time preparing themselves for the surgery itself.

Of course, putting in time to find the right doctor is important. Patients should choose a surgeon with the skill, experience, and personality that align with their particular needs. I recommend choosing a surgeon that is a *subspecialist*. Subspecialization means that the vast majority of the surgeon's practice is focused on a particular type of surgery. I am a subspecialist in total joint replacement, and, as such, nearly 100 percent of my practice consists of performing hip and knee replacements.

Additionally, patients are wise to choose a surgeon who performs a great many operations in the subspecialty. In the case of total joint replacement, this means a minimum of hundreds of joint replacements per year. This is not simply my opinion. Many scientific studies demonstrate improved patient outcomes and decreased complications with high-volume subspecialists. Likewise, studies show that patients are wise to choose hospitals that perform a large number of surgical cases; these hospitals routinely outperform lower-volume hospitals, particularly with regard to complication rates.

However, as I stated earlier, choosing the right surgeon (and hospital) is only 10 percent of the equation. The other 90 percent is actually you! As an analogy, consider a person who decides to get in shape by joining a gym. That person could join the cheapest, no-frills facility, and with the right expectations, mindset, and execution achieve remarkable fitness gains. On the other hand, that same person could join the most expensive gym in town with the newest exercise equipment and the "best," most sought-after trainers. However, if unwilling to put in the time and effort, he or she will not shed a single pound of fat or gain an ounce of muscle and will consequently be dissatisfied with the results.

The difference then, whether it be working out or recovering from orthopedic surgery, is not necessarily the trainer, the equipment, or the surgeon (assuming you choose a competent and experienced one). The difference is you.

The recipe for success is three-pronged: it involves having the right expectations, the right mindset, and the right execution of the recovery plan. Expectations drive everything, including mindset and execution. It is my experience in having treated thousands of patients for hip and knee replacements that patients with appropriate expectations are generally the most satisfied following surgery. Patients who expect to do well, who expect to go home (rather than to rehab), who expect to be independent, and who expect to achieve pain relief usually do just that.

A small aside will illustrate the importance of expectations. There are a variety of ways in which patients make it into my clinic. For some, it is at the referral from their primary doctor. Others heard about me through a friend or family member. Some simply call our office and ask for the first available doctor to see them for their hip or knee problem. However, a certain percentage of patients specifically seek me out for the special minimally invasive knee replacement that I perform. Some even come from other states for this procedure. It is my distinct observation that this last group of patients—those who are specifically seeking a minimally invasive procedure and a faster recovery—do the best.

Why? Because they *expect* to. They expect that minimally invasive surgery will give them an advantage in their recovery. (I certainly believe it too.) They expect that they will have improved pain control, and they expect that they will do better than their friends with standard knee replacements. And over and over again they do. The mind is a powerful force in the healing process.

How are expectations set? Clearly, patients come in with some preconceived notions. Some are realistic, some are less so. Sometimes patients have no idea what to expect. It is thus imperative that, before the surgery, patients discuss their goals and plan their postoperative recovery. These issues are covered in detail in this book.

The second element for successful surgery is mindset. Whereas expectations can be shaped by proper education (via this book, your surgeon, friends, family, hospital classes, online resources, etc.), mindset comes from within. Total joint replacement is elective surgery aimed at improving quality of life; arthritis is not a life-threatening condition. As such, patients should not proceed with total joint surgery until they have the appropriate mindset. Very simply, that mindset should be:

1. I have exhausted the nonoperative options to treat my arthritis.
2. My arthritis is seriously affecting the quality of my life.
3. I am physically and mentally ready for this operation.
4. I am willing to do everything I can to maximize my recovery.

Until this mindset is established, I do not think patients are ready to embark on this journey. Of particular significance is becoming mentally ready, which means assigning your recovery a high priority in your daily life for the next few months.

With the appropriate expectations and mindset, execution of the recovery plan becomes relatively straightforward. This includes reporting and actively managing postoperative pain, diligently performing physical therapy and prescribed exercises, and maintaining a positive attitude. It is also important to communicate your needs and concerns with your surgeon, primary doctor, and physical therapist, and to do everything you can to maximize your postoperative recovery and long-term outcome.

Keep in mind that complete recovery from a major orthopedic surgery takes time. A good rule of thumb is that after an operation such as a hip or knee replacement, patients are 75 percent recovered by six weeks, 90 percent by three months, and fully recovered by a year. It simply takes time for the body to heal itself and for the inflammatory response to run its course. Proper execution is a long-term endeavor that requires a healthy dose of patience.

If you are reading this book, chances are you are on the right path. In many ways, you already have an advantage. Elizabeth Kaufmann has created an excellent resource to appropriately align your expectations, hone your mindset, and empower you to properly execute your plan. Remember, 90 percent is up to you.

—Jared Foran, MD
Director of Joint Replacement Surgery
OrthoColorado Hospital and St. Anthony Hospital
Lakewood, Colorado

Introduction

What You Know Can Only Help You

One morning I was teaching the physical therapy portion of a class for prospective total knee and hip patients. The seminar was called Joint Class, and all of the attendees had either signed up for surgery or were accompanying family members who had signed up. The hospital was a new, ultra-high-tech facility called OrthoColorado in west Denver, specializing in planned orthopedic surgeries.[1] As one of two physical therapists who inaugurated the rehabilitation program at this posh forty-eight-bed hospital when it opened in 2010, I was a frequent presenter at joint class. The nurse leading it wanted me to limit my talk to fifteen minutes, something I was rarely capable of doing, because there was so much material to cover and people asked so many questions. I was clarifying something about the post-hospital recovery, when a fit-looking man in his late forties sitting in the back raised his hand.

"Do you think I will be able to ride my mountain bike within two weeks after my knee replacement?" he asked with an expectant look.

I stared at him, shocked by the wishful thinking his question revealed. But I've learned over the years that patients can be woefully uninformed about the realities of joint surgery. And no question should be off limits. A number of patients in other classes had asked more intimate questions, such as how soon after their hip or spine surgery could they have sex, and in what positions. Others ask when they can drive or when they can return to work.

I knew the cyclist would hate my answer. I, too, ride a mountain bike in the Colorado foothills and understand how hard it can be to give up a favorite activity. But at least the sacrifice—and this is true of most of the activities people love—is only temporary. Without the surgery, the option of playing tennis or skiing or golfing, or whatever activity or sport is too painful now, may be lost forever.

"You could ride a stationary bike indoors, or put your bike on a trainer, the first week you're home from surgery," I replied. "It's a great way to get your knee bending. But I think it will take at least six to eight weeks before you'll be able to ride outside on hills or technical terrain." Even this answer was pushing the limits of what Stephen Colbert would call "truthiness."

He frowned.

"If it's going to take that long, I may just cancel the surgery," he said.

Of course, it wasn't my fault he was disappointed, but I felt badly and wanted the opportunity to talk to him further and try to explain. I wanted to say if his knee already hurt so much that he couldn't ride, the surgery would give him the option of riding again, but not within two weeks. If he could still ride now without debilitating knee pain, maybe he wasn't ready for the surgery. But I didn't get the chance to talk to him at all, because the class was rushed, and then he was gone.

Patient satisfaction is important, and our health-care delivery system, starting with the hospital setting, has begun to take it much more seriously.[2] Your feedback about your experience carries more weight now than you might imagine. While the reasons for this are complex, there is a clear economic incentive to make patients happier, happier with the service they receive in the hospital, and happier with the ultimate outcome of their surgery. A small percentage of the payment to hospitals and physicians by Medicare, the primary insurance for people 65 and over, is already tied to patient satisfaction. This trend, the correlation of payments to outcomes and patient satisfaction, is expected to grow in the future.

At the same time, while patient satisfaction carries greater weight, orthopedics has become a ripe testing ground for policy makers to investigate how to reduce health-care costs.[3] This combination—the drive to cut costs juxtaposed with the very real attempt to make care more patient-centered—can pose an interesting challenge for you as you try to identify your best options. The new focus on consumerism means that you have choices. You should take them seriously, just as you would if you were buying a house or a car. If you carefully consider what's best for you, you are much more likely to be satisfied with the end product.

YOUR SURGERY COMPANION

The operations covered in this book include knee and hip replacement—which account for more than one million surgeries per year in the United States—plus shoulder replacement, ankle replacement, and spinal fusion surgery—which together account for another half million or more.[4]

If your surgery includes a hospital stay, my hope is that you read this book before the big day, then pack it in your hospital bag. The material is presented in the same chronological order as your experience, and you can quickly identify the specifics of your diagnosis, skipping over the procedures and chapters that don't apply.

Chapter 1 encourages you to take time to **choose your surgeon wisely** and gives you tips on how to do so.

Chapter 2 explains your **pre-op tasks**: lining up help at home, learning the prohibited movements for your diagnosis, mastering basic exercises, and, if necessary, modifying your home.

Chapter 3 is dedicated to helping people who live alone **plan for the post-op recovery** period.

In Chapter 4, you'll get a **crash course on hospital equipment**—all those quirky and noisy lines, tubes, and machines that will be attached to you following surgery.

Chapter 5 identifies and describes the **role of the different clinicians, caregivers, and service people** you will encounter during your hospital stay.

Chapter 6 emphasizes the importance of **sharing your fears, social habits, and any mental-health issues** that could affect your recovery with the hospital staff.

Chapter 7 gives you a detailed description of the different kinds of **medications** used to address pain, and how the side effects of these drugs are managed.

Chapter 8 provides a general framework for the **rehabilitation therapy** you will likely receive for each diagnosis, starting in the hospital and progressing into the weeks after you leave.

Chapter 9 explains how **hospital culture** has changed and describes how both providers and patients are more accountable.

Chapter 10 illuminates the importance of the **discharge** process and offers a list of the things you and your caregiver should know before you go.

Throughout the text, medical terms placed in italics are defined in the glossary at the end of the book.

What you learn will build your confidence, decrease the apprehension you may feel about your impending surgery, and help you navigate this challenging experience with greater ease and control. As an added benefit, much of the material in this book will also help you find your way through other medical experiences, including any hospital stay.

While knee replacement may win the prize for "toughest recovery," none of the operations covered in this book are a quick fix. Your new body part should feel better in time, but it won't duplicate the pristine original. Healing takes more time than you may expect and requires a strong dose of patience. But if pain, stiffness, or disability have interfered with your life, and you've tried conservative measures such as therapy, injections, and anti-inflammatory drugs to little or only temporary avail, and the list of things you can do is continually shrinking, joint replacement and spine surgery are restorative, life-enriching options that can eliminate all or nearly all of the pain. What you have to accept is that recovery is a biological phenomenon, and there are limits to what you can do to speed up the process.

The good news is that the quality of each of these surgeries keeps improving—with smaller, tissue-sparing incisions, better surgical techniques, and shorter anesthesia times—and the quality of the implants continues to evolve. As long as you're proactive and prepared to do some work before and after surgery, you can recover fully and get your life back. One inspiring example is the man in his sixties who sent our therapy department at OrthoColorado a picture of himself on top of one of Colorado's many fourteen-thousand-foot peaks. These peaks pose a significant challenge to anyone, even a hiker with good knees. He was wearing shorts, hiking boots, and a big smile. The scar on one of his knees was barely discernible in the photograph.

"Here I am, six months after my knee replacement," the caption read. We displayed the picture in our therapy gym, hoping it would inspire other patients as much as it pleased us. He had made a steep ascent at high altitude to reach his personal goal, reaching that mountaintop. There is no possible way he could have done it two weeks after surgery. But he did it after six months. And isn't that what matters in the long run?

WHY I'M WRITING THIS BOOK

During my seventeen-year tenure as a physical therapist, I came to love orthopedics. I repeatedly saw how the interventions and skills I learned and shared with orthopedic patients made a dramatic and immediate impact in the quality of their lives. I've worked with thousands of orthopedic patients in the hospital, in their homes, and, to a lesser degree, in the outpatient setting. Many are fellow baby boomers. I've taught them how to walk when they didn't believe they could, and I've given countless pep talks reassuring them that their spirit, strength, and energy would eventually return. It was immensely rewarding to help people recover after surgery. And most orthopedic surgeons would agree that at least some physical therapy is vital to a full recovery from major elective orthopedic surgery.

Another fulfilling part of my work was the experience of observing how even a small amount of preoperative education, in the form of joint class, made a big difference in the way patients coped with the aftereffects of surgery. The ones who understood the most about what to expect were always the calmest patients, the ones who seemed to be in control of their situation.

At this time, most specialty hospitals do provide some sort of a class, and I highly recommend that you attend. At OrthoColorado, we taught classes for knee, hip, and spine patients, and I frequently heard afterward from those who attended our classes how helpful they were and how difficult it would have been to go through surgery without them. I believe it's also best when each group of patients can have its own class. Shoulder patients should not have to sit through a knee class, and hip patients should not have to sit through a spine class. Classes require a dedicated team effort and a certain commitment of resources, and there is no uniform way that hospitals provide this education. Some do a better job than others.

The Hospital for Special Surgery (HSS) in New York pioneered knee replacement surgery in the 1970s, and it is consistently ranked as the number one orthopedic hospital in *U.S. News and World Report*. The dedicated orthopedic staff at HSS took the concept of joint class a step further.[5] A study by Rupali Joshi, PT, PhD, took 126 patients planning a hip or knee replacement, and randomly divided them into two groups.[6] One group attended a joint class and received a written manual. The second group received those services plus a thirty-minute, one-on-one session with a physical therapist. Patients in the second group were "better prepared to leave the hospital after surgery and were overall more satisfied with the preoperative education they received." They also required fewer hospital physical therapy visits for a safe discharge home. Of the patients in the first group, 70 percent said they would have benefited from more education.[7]

Not everybody can go to HSS for orthopedic surgery. But wouldn't it be great if other orthopedic hospitals offered one-on-one education with a physical therapist before surgery? To my knowledge, most hospitals do not offer this level of upfront service, even though studies have shown that it helps patients. Patient-centered care is on the rise, but it still has a long way to go.

Another study showed that total knee and hip patients who received one to two preoperative physical therapy sessions, called *prehabilitation*, incurred 29 percent less in costs on postoperative therapy, including skilled nursing facilities and home health services. Doesn't it make sense that informed and prepared patients recover better, feel better, and spend less time and money than uninformed and unprepared ones?

I believe that all patients deserve the opportunity to reap the benefits that education can offer, and I aim to give you the vital information you need for your specific joint replacement or spine surgery. I will help you shape your expectations and guide you to making informed decisions about a significant event in your life.

My hope is that the lessons shared here will help you feel in greater control of your experience. If hospitals are a mystery to you, they should be less intimidating and more transparent after you read this book. You will become the patient who plans ahead and makes adjustments at home before surgery, who handles the hospital stay with calmness and grace, and who learns to accept a reasonable amount of pain.

Recovery is a whole-body process; it's not just about the surgery site. Recovery happens in your cells and your blood and your heart and your psyche. The reward of a healthier, stronger body will take time, but when you know what to expect and how to manage the process, you will discover your hard work paying off. All you have to do is get involved. Take ownership of the things you can control. Embrace the coming transformation in your life, like the former patient standing victoriously on that Colorado summit. Whatever mountain you need to climb, it will be waiting for you when you're ready.

Chapter 1

Choosing Your Surgeon

I am often surprised by how little people know about their surgeon. But nothing could be more important than your comfort level with this individual. While this book will focus primarily on what to do after you have a surgeon, here are a few things to consider when choosing one.

When you have an elective surgery, as opposed to an emergency, there is plenty of time to research and choose your doctor. You want to know as much as you can about the individual physician, not just the practice. You also want to know something about the hospital setting.

When you are looking for a doctor, it is important to remember that you don't need to commit to the first one that is available. Meet with several candidates, and pay attention if your first impressions leave you wary. You will have at least a one-year-long relationship with whichever surgeon you choose. Don't be embarrassed about seeking a second opinion; the doctor's ego can handle it. If there is a question about what needs to be done, a caring surgeon will be the one to recommend getting a second opinion, preferably from another practice.

My husband found himself in this predicament when he needed a knee replacement. Ernie had exhausted the conservative treatment options and had reached the point that even sitting in the car for more than a few minutes was causing more aching pain than he could tolerate. His primary surgeon thought there was a small chance he could get by with a partial replacement because most of the cartilage loss had occurred on just one side of his knee. In addition, at 57, Ernie was somewhat young for a total knee. But an MRI revealed that his anterior cruciate ligament (ACL), a vital ligament to protect the knee from hyperextending, or over-straightening, was shredded, likely from a high school football injury. Due to the ACL issue, the doctor believed that a partial replacement would not provide adequate stability in the knee, but recommended a second opinion, outside the practice. The second surgeon agreed that a total replacement was needed. Ernie returned to his primary surgeon, who performed the operation. Afterward, the doctor came up to the floor where I was working, told me everything had gone well, and said, "He definitely needed the total." Without a second opinion, Ernie would have questioned whether he had done the right thing. Now he knows he did, and the knee is working beautifully and without pain.

Sometimes there are other less invasive and more conservative options—such as therapy, injections, medications, and bracing—than a joint replacement, and these are always worth exploring. The same is true of spine fusion surgery. A consult with another expert prior to a major elective orthopedic surgery is usually covered by insurance. Ask your primary care physician or a physical therapist you know for a recommendation. Ask your friends and colleagues as well. Don't rush.

My bias as a patient and physical therapist is toward choosing a surgeon who performs a large number of the same procedure I need—a specialist as opposed to a generalist. I would prefer a surgeon who has a great track record and performs more than three hundred knee replacements annually over one who performs thirty. I would also prefer a specialty center, where the entire staff is trained in and dedicated to orthopedics, to avoid receiving care by nurses, for example, who may not be as familiar with the orthopedic movement precautions for a spine, shoulder, or hip patient, or the nuances and side effects of each pain medication. Research shows that outcomes are better among individual surgeons who perform a high volume of these surgeries, and in the hospitals where they perform them.[8]

Personally, I would also like a physician who listens well and has a good bedside manner. Does he make eye contact and give you time to ask questions? Does he ask about the severity of your pain and the specific activities that bother you? Does he consider you as a whole person with a profession and responsibilities at home, who may also be passionate about a hobby or a sport? Does he perform a thorough physical exam of the body part that hurts in addition to looking at your imaging exams or films? Does he explain, using a model or an x-ray of your affected body part, where the problem lies and how he intends to address it? A single visit can give you a good idea of his concern for you as a person.

You can look up your potential surgeon and hospital on a number of websites; including ProPublica.org (check the Surgeon Scorecard under Data/Patient Safety), vitals.com, healthgrades.com, and Medicare.gov/hospitalcompare. ProPublica's database shows individual rates of complications for surgeons by name and also for their hospitals. If you do some sleuthing, you will get a good idea how your surgeon compares with others in your region. It is also important to check the safety data on your selected hospital. In most cases, you will find that the most highly rated surgeons operate in the most highly rated hospitals.

One caveat about databases: a surgeon who takes on sicker or more complex patients may appear to have inferior outcomes, but these may reflect the patients' compromised preoperative health rather than the surgeon's skills. Feel free to ask your surgeon about the procedures he or she most frequently performs, and whether the patients are similar or different from you in age and health status.

Once you find the right surgeon for you, make sure you fully understand the upcoming procedure—but remember that is only part of the whole picture. The surgeon is focused on the surgery, which is as it should be. The surgery is the centerpiece of this undertaking, the part that you have entrusted to a highly trained expert. The surgeon should explain your procedure in terms you can understand, including the type of implant, how long surgery will take, details about the approach and the incision, and options for anesthesia.

But the surgeon will not tell you how to prepare your living space, what activities and exercises to practice ahead of time (although some may do so), what equipment you will need, what the hospital stay is like, and what kind of help you will need at home. Frankly, surgeons are not trained at teaching these things, and most of the time they are simply too busy. Apart from the surgery itself, everything else that needs to happen in the weeks before and after the operation is ultimately up to you.

By all means, if your hospital offers a preoperative class for your diagnosis, you should attend. Some surgeons have made these classes mandatory. Carefully read all literature or pamphlets provided by your surgeon's office. And whether or not you have a class to attend, be sure to refer to this book for greater detail and key strategies for navigating the entire experience, ranging from the presurgical period to the far side of recovery.

Chapter 2

Getting Ready for Surgery

You are likely feeling some apprehension about your upcoming surgery. Maybe it feels like the big unknown, and you have no control. Or maybe you think that finally, somebody is going to "fix" your pain.

I will disabuse you of both of these ideas. The big unknown actually consists of a small time period, the few hours during which you are anesthetized and then in recovery. The rest of the time, before and after surgery, you actually have a great deal of influence over what transpires. Second, I would warn against the passive belief that the surgeon is going to "fix" you so all your pain will go away. It's true that he is going to replace a damaged body part, but your body is not a machine. It would be more accurate to say that the quality of the pain will change. Some total hip patients report immediate relief after surgery from the grinding pain they felt, replaced by an incisional pain, which is tolerable and temporary. Regardless of your diagnosis, you will be living with some pain for a certain amount of time after surgery.

I will give you a primer of information in this chapter about the things you need to know before surgery. If you want to feel less anxious, it helps to feel in control. Before you can feel in control, you need knowledge—knowledge of your affected body parts and condition, an understanding of what to expect in the hospital, what equipment you may need and how to set up your home, and the things you should and shouldn't do after surgery. Once you achieve a better understanding of your situation, you may be able to let go of some of your apprehension. You may be able to take that visceral fear that creeps up and spin it into something different, perhaps even something like excitement. You may be able to say to yourself in pre-op, *Okay, I trust my surgical team to take good care of me, and I've done everything I can to prepare for this, so now I'm just going to relax.*

It is going to take some work on your part. I think you will feel more empowered if you do some homework. It won't take long, but you should start as soon as you can, at least a month before surgery. The homework will be very easy, because I am going to give you the answers.

BODY PARTS AND PROSTHESES

A quick overview of your affected joint's anatomy and the proposed procedure will improve your understanding and your ability to communicate physical sensations and pain levels to your providers. Below are general descriptions of the joints and operations covered in this book. While your specific surgery may be different—you could have a partial rather than total replacement of the knee, hip, or shoulder, for example—knowledge of your anatomy will help.

Knee Replacement

A knee replacement is actually a resurfacing of the diseased parts. The lower end of the thighbone, or *femur*, is trimmed of rough bone and fitted with a metal cover called the femoral component. The top of the shinbone, the *tibia*, is smoothed and subsequently covered with a flat plate that includes a stem. This is the tibial component. A strong polyethylene (plastic) piece called a spacer is locked into the top of the tibial component to provide a smooth gliding surface with the new surface of the femur. The underside of the kneecap, or *patella*, is trimmed of rough cartilage and fitted with a small piece of polyethylene, often called a button and shaped like a dome, which provides a smooth interface with the other two parts. The top (skin side) of the kneecap, not shown below, remains intact.

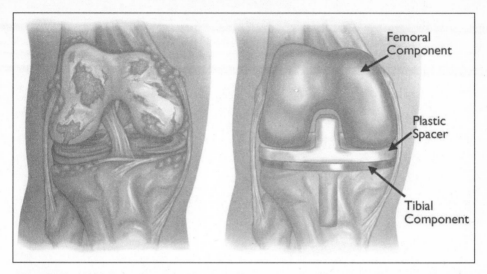

An arthritic right knee from the front (left) and a replaced knee (right). Kneecap not shown. Reproduced with permission from OrthoInfo. ©American Academy of Orthopaedic Surgeons. http://orthoinfo.aaos.org.

Hip Replacement

The hip joint is the union of the ball-shaped top of the thighbone, or *femoral head*, with the socket in the pelvis, called the *acetabulum*. During a total hip surgery, the femoral head is removed, along with the short neck below it. The head is replaced with a ball-shaped piece, which sits on top of a metal neck that is connected to a metal stem. The ball is made of metal or ceramic. This stem is fitted down into a hollow part of the thighbone. The acetabulum is cleaned of damaged tissue and replaced with a prosthetic metal socket, also called a cup, that is secured to the pelvis with or without screws. A liner, shaped like an upside-down bowl and made of plastic, ceramic, or metal, is fitted over the new femoral head to serve as a buffer, like cartilage, and to promote a smooth interface with the new socket. Metal-on-metal surfaces have shown to be controversial, and a good question to ask your surgeon is what materials are used in your prosthesis and why they were chosen.

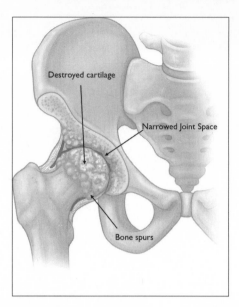

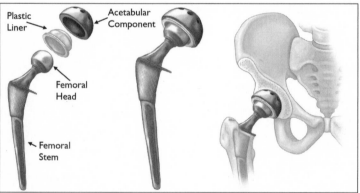

An arthritic right hip with destroyed cartilage on the femoral head as well as on the acetabulum (above). Components of a hip replacement (above left and center) and a replaced hip (above right). Reproduced with permission from OrthoInfo. ©American Academy of Orthopaedic Surgeons. http://orthoinfo.aaos.org.

Total Shoulder Replacement

The shoulder, like the hip, is a ball and socket joint. The round top of the arm bone, called the *humeral head*, fits into a shallow socket on the *scapula* called the *glenoid cavity*. The collarbone, or *clavicle*, connects the top of the scapula to the *sternum* and plays a role in stabilizing the arm. In a conventional shoulder replacement, the humeral head is removed and replaced with a metallic ball and a stem that fits down into the upper arm bone. The glenoid cavity is surgically trimmed of rough cartilage and covered with a plastic socket.

In a reverse total shoulder, the new components are reversed. The round humeral head is cut off and replaced with a plastic concave cup that fits into the upper arm, and the glenoid is fitted with a convex metal ball that is secured with screws into the cavity on the scapula. This technique has proven successful for people who have lost function of their rotator cuff muscles, as it allows the deltoid muscles on top of the arm to compensate and control the arm.

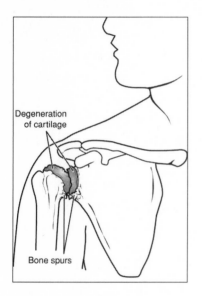

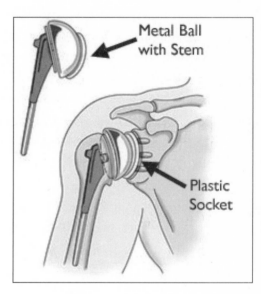

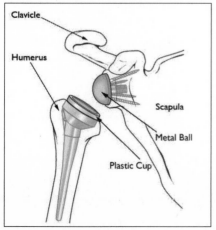

An arthritic right shoulder (above left), a conventional shoulder replacement in place (above), and the components of a reverse total shoulder replacement (left). Reproduced with permission from OrthoInfo. ©American Academy of Orthopaedic Surgeons. http://orthoinfo.aaos.org.

Spine Fusion Surgery

The purpose of a fusion surgery is to eliminate pain originating in movement of two or more vertebrae in the spine by welding those vertebrae together. The *cervical spine* has seven vertebrae, the *thoracic spine* has twelve, all connected to the ribs, the *lumbar spine* has five, and the *sacrum* has two. Fusions are often performed on the most naturally mobile segments in the neck and the low back. When movement at these segments is eliminated by a fusion, the adjacent segments tend to compensate by moving more.

Whether the surgeon approaches the neck or lumbar spine from the back (posterior) or front (anterior), or the side (lateral) in some lumbar cases, the basic components of a fusion surgery are similar. When two lumbar vertebrae are fused, the disk is removed from between them, and a bone graft, packed inside a cage, is inserted in its place. The graft can consist of your own bone, taken from the pelvis in a separate incision, a cadaver bone (allograft), or a synthetic material. In a cervical-spine fusion with an anterior approach, a device called a spacer is used instead of a cage and is made from allograft bone, plastic, or metal. No spacer or cage is used in a posterior approach.

In any given spine fusion procedure, the surgeon may use screws, plates, rods, or wires to secure the vertebrae together and promote an optimal union between them. Sometimes fusion surgeries are performed on more

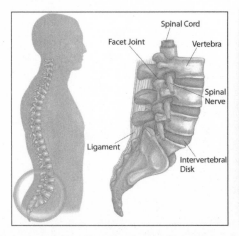
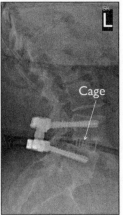

Normal spine anatomy (above) and a lumbar cage in place with two screws to stabilize the fusion (above right). Reproduced with permission from OrthoInfo. ©American Academy of Orthopaedic Surgeons. http://orthoinfo.aaos.org.

than one level, such as L4–L5 and L5–S1. This is a fusion of the fourth and fifth lumbar vertebrae, and the fifth lumbar with the first sacral vertebrae.

Ankle Replacement

The ankle joint contains three parts: the lower end of the shinbone, or tibia; the lower end of the *fibula*, the outer leg bone; and the bone at the top of the foot called the *talus*, which sits between them (and underneath the tibia, which arches over it). The junction of these bones allows for pointing and flexing the foot. In an ankle replacement, the surgeon approaches the foot from the front or the outside. The arthritic surfaces of the tibia, the primary weight-bearing bone in the lower leg, and the talus are cleared of their damaged cartilage and trimmed to allow room for the implant.

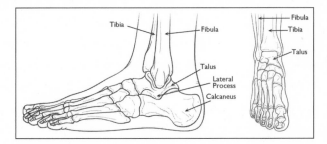

Normal foot anatomy from the side (left) and the front (right). The union of the talus and the low ends of the tibia and fibula make up the ankle joint. Reproduced with permission from OrthoInfo. ©American Academy of Orthopaedic Surgeons. http://orthoinfo.aaos.org.

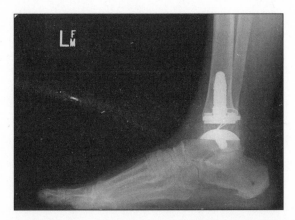

A replaced ankle. Reproduced with permission from Ishikawa SN, Gause LN: "Immunologic rheumatic disorders of the foot and ankle." *Orthopaedic Knowledge Online Journal* 2012; Volume 10 Number 8. Accessed February 2015.

The implant consists of two main parts. The upper or tibial component of the implant is made of a metal top with a stem and a polyethylene spacer below. This spacer glides on top of the second piece underneath, called the talar component, which is made of metal.

FOUR KEY CONCEPTS

Here are four topics to read about and give serious thought to before your surgery: **Length of Stay**, **Precautions**, **Home Safety**, and **Early Exercises and Activities**. After I define them, I will discuss each one further under separate sections for each type of surgery.

Length of Stay is the number of nights in the hospital insurance typically covers for your diagnosis. If you dislike hospitals and can't wait to get home to your own bed, you will be delighted to know that you may spend just one night in the hospital after your shoulder or ankle replacement and even after your hip or knee replacement. But if you prefer having professionals take care of you as long as possible, rather than relying on a spouse or family member, you may be surprised at the brevity of your stay.

The hospital stay for each of these diagnoses is trending shorter—one to two nights in some cases—and you may not feel ready to go home that soon. This means that you and your family carry a greater responsibility for postoperative care than ever before, including hands-on care. (This trend belongs to the cost-cutting part of US health-care policy, but it is also healthier to get out of the hospital.) Don't be lulled into thinking your surgeon can bend the rules and keep you in the hospital an extra day because of your close relationship with him. There has to be a specific medical reason to keep you that warrants a hospital staff's expertise and oversight.

People in the hospital do care about your well-being and should not send you home until you are medically ready. If you really need more time, you should get it. The last thing a hospital wants is for you to be readmitted; this counts as a black mark against the hospital and can reduce its reimbursement. But the reason for keeping you has to be a medical one that pertains to your current health status, such as a heart rhythm abnormality. You won't get an extra day in the hospital because the friend or relative staying with you can't get into town on the day of your scheduled discharge, or because your husband is on a business trip. This is why you need to be prepared.

Call your insurance company before surgery to ask about the length of stay for your procedure. If you don't get a definitive answer, call the orthopedic case manager or clinical care coordinator at your hospital and have your insurance information handy. It is a good idea to acquaint yourself with the case manager or clinical care coordinator—some, but not all, hospitals have a person who will call every patient in advance—because this is the person who will oversee your discharge plan once you are admitted, the person who will ask who is taking you home and staying with you and for how long (see chapter 3). Case managers at my hospital called patients ahead of surgery to discuss discharge planning to help make sure everyone was on the same page.

Knowing your length of stay facilitates planning for the help you will need at home, especially if someone is traveling from out of town to care for you. It's best to plan for the quoted length of stay from the insurance company or case manager, rather than hope for extra days. If you end up needing more time, your caregiver can learn more about your specific needs by coming to the hospital the day before discharge.

Precautions are discussed here in two parts. First are restrictions on how much weight you can put on the newly operated body part. If you are having an ankle replacement, for instance, you will be *non-weight bearing* (NWB) on that foot for a number of weeks, meaning you may not step on it. You will need to use crutches, a walker, a knee scooter or a wheelchair, or some combination of these devices. If you know you will be non-weight bearing, it's much better to figure out which devices work best for you and learn to use them before surgery rather than waiting until afterward.

If you are having a knee or hip replacement, you will need one or more of these assistive devices as well, but you will be allowed to bear weight on the new body part, a status called *weight bearing as tolerated* (WBAT). Exceptions occur in knee or hip patients if the quality of the bone is compromised or if a fracture occurs during surgery. If you are told that you may only put partial weight on the operated leg, ask the surgeon the reason. Don't settle for a surrogate's response, such as, "Because the surgeon says so." Spine fusion patients should be WBAT even if a bone graft is harvested from the pelvis.

Here's a quick tutorial on *assistive devices* such as walkers, crutches, and canes. A *front-wheeled walker* (FWW) is the device preferred by physical therapists for the majority of patients immediately following knee or hip replacement. The reason is that it allows you to transfer as much body weight as you need to from your lower body to your upper body and onto the walker, via your arms. The front-wheeled walker also facilitates the return to normal walking pattern as you gain strength and confidence.

In the beginning, you will push the walker forward, take a step with your surgical leg while pushing down on the walker with your arms, then follow with your stronger leg. Therapists call this a *step-to* pattern: you step forward with one foot and bring the other one to meet it. It looks like a limp. But in normal walking, you *step through*, bringing the rear foot past the front one. Many people cannot do a step-through pattern initially after knee or hip surgery, due to discomfort. If you are having a lumbar spine fusion, and you have one leg that is weaker or hurts more, a front-wheeled walker will help significantly in the early stages after surgery.

A *standard walker*, one without wheels, doesn't allow for normalizing your walking pattern because you have to pick it up with each step. A *four-wheeled walker* doesn't give you enough support for pushing down, as the wheels not only roll forward, but also rotate, turning sideways. A front-wheeled walker is covered by insurance (as of this writing), but a four-wheeled walker is not.

If you have a borrowed or second-hand front-wheeled walker, here's how to assess it for fit and suitability. First, make sure it is solid and does not wobble. Stand up straight inside the walker and see if you can adjust its height (each of the four feet has notches) to bring the handles to the level of your wrists. There should be a slight bend in your elbows when you push down on the handles; you shouldn't have to reach down, nor should your shoulders creep up toward your ears. Second, make sure the wheels actually roll; if one is stuck, clean out any dirt in the mechanism and spray it with a lubricant such as WD-40. If that doesn't work, don't use it. A bad wheel can ruin your day.

A pair of crutches is sometimes the device of choice for younger patients, especially those who have used them before. You may bring your own crutches (or walker) to the hospital, or have your companion bring them to your room after surgery.

Fitting crutches is slightly more difficult than fitting a walker. First, when you stand up straight, there should be a three-finger-width gap between your armpit and the top of the crutch; adjust this height first. (Note that crutches often have heights marked on them, but these can be misleading.) The reason for the distance between your armpit and the top of the crutch is to prevent the crutch from sticking as you move forward, and also to encourage you not to rest on your armpits. Bearing down through your armpits when you walk is incorrect, as this can put pressure on the *axillary nerve*, which can lead to tingling, numbness, and weakness in the front of the shoulder. Second, the hand pieces should come to your wrists, just as with a walker. When walking with crutches, hug them close to your body and put your weight through the hand pieces. The correct walking patterns are the same as with walkers, starting with step-to after surgery and progressing to step-through.

A cane should also be fitted to your wrist level. Nearly every knee and hip patient will need a cane, first for using on stairs and then for using on level surfaces as you progress from the walker. The correct way to carry the cane is on the strong, nonsurgical side. This is because humans have what's called a *reciprocal gait* (walking) pattern: when one leg advances, so does the opposite arm. If you have your right knee replaced, you carry the cane in your left hand.

Step forward with the right foot as you simultaneously place the cane in front on your left. Notice how some of the weight from your right leg is transferred to your left arm. If you carry the cane incorrectly, on the surgical side, you will waddle like a duck or like actor Hugh Laurie when he played Dr. Gregory House.[9]

Insurance will typically cover one of these three walking devices. A front-wheeled walker, if billed through insurance, costs the most ($100 or more), followed by crutches (roughly $50), then a cane ($15 to $20). Your insurance policy should have a section on durable medical equipment (DME); call if you don't see what's covered. If you are having a knee, hip, or lumbar spine surgery and if you think you will need a walker after reading up on your specific surgery, it makes sense to buy a cane for using on stairs, and let insurance pay for the walker. Canes are available in most drug stores; for other equipment, you might check a medical supply store.

If you have to pay for equipment out of pocket, you may also be able to find it at a charitable outlet or a thrift store. A new front-wheeled walker is available online for as little as thirty dollars.

Wheelchairs are only covered in rare cases, as they are not usually necessary after any of these surgeries (unless you are already using one), with the possible exception of an ankle replacement. In that case, a rental wheelchair may be covered, but it will need to be ordered by the hospital staff after a therapist or doctor has determined a need for it.

A knee scooter, also called a knee walker, can appeal to post-op total ankle patients. You can rest your surgical leg and foot on the scooter, parallel to the floor, and propel the scooter with your good leg. While it looks easy, it can be tricky to use and requires good balance and agility. My internist used one to navigate around his office after rupturing his Achilles tendon. A scooter can be rented or purchased, but it is rarely covered by insurance. Some people have good luck finding a used knee scooter online from a site such as Craigslist.

The second type of precaution pertains to specific movements that you will need to avoid with your diagnosis. Hip replacement patients have hip precautions, shoulder patients have shoulder precautions, and spine patients have spine precautions. Not only is it best to memorize these in advance, but I suggest thinking about how they will affect your ability to perform everyday activities such as getting dressed, picking up things from the floor, or getting up from a toilet or low chair. See more about precautions in your specific procedure section below.

Home Safety pertains to functioning safely at home after your surgery. It helps to imagine exactly how you will be moving and walking. Everything will take more time.

Things to consider: Do you have obstacles that could cause you to trip, such as throw rugs, pet toys, or electrical cords? Do you need to go upstairs to your bedroom after your ankle replacement or is there another place where you can sleep? Many post-op patients, regardless of the diagnosis, set up a sleeping space on the ground floor to save energy. Do the stairs leading into your house have a railing? When you consider home safety, also think about it in terms of your precautions. Will you be able to sit on a regular-height toilet after your hip replacement (if you have precautions), or will you need a riser or a raised seat with a frame for pushing yourself up? How will you step in and out of your bathtub? If you are right-handed and are having a right shoulder replacement, how will you compensate for all the things you do with your right hand?

If you have a dog, think about having someone care for it, or at least walk it, while you recuperate. Also, make sure you have adequate traction in your shower or tub to prevent slipping, use nightlights in the bathroom, and do as much as you can to make and freeze meals ahead of time or accept help from friends and family for such tasks as vacuuming, grocery shopping, and doing laundry.

Early Exercises and Activities will be initiated in the hospital for knee, hip, and most shoulder patients. While these exercises are basic and simple, they aren't quite so easy to learn or to execute after surgery. Indeed, these simple activities can flummox people who haven't done them before, especially those who get spacey on narcotics. Well-prepared patients, therefore, routinely learn and practice their basic exercises in the comfort of home, before surgery. Bending your knee and tightening your *quadriceps* (front of thigh) or buttock muscles will feel different after surgery, but at least you will know what you are doing and why.

Neck and back patients will not be given exercises in the hospital and will not start outpatient therapy until many weeks later. The main recommended activity for post-surgical spine patients is walking, and unless it is prohibitively painful, it's a smart idea to begin a walking program before the operation.

Ankle replacement patients will not be given specific exercises in the hospital, either, except possibly to wiggle the toes frequently; the ankle itself will be immobilized in a splint. You will be prescribed outpatient therapy after the wound has healed, to begin building range of motion and strength in the foot and ankle. However, if you are having an ankle replacement, remember that you will be non-weight bearing for a period of approximately six weeks. If you do not plan to be wheelchair-bound during this time, you will need to learn to use a walker or crutches on level surfaces and one crutch and a railing on stairs. If you are not young or not an athlete and are not accustomed to crutches, now would be a good time to practice using them, before surgery. See the ankle replacement section for a description of exercises to help strengthen the muscles you will recruit and rely on when using crutches.

A general note about fitness: it's helpful and important to get into the best shape you possibly can before surgery (as well as to eat a nutritious diet). If your ability to walk is limited, try swimming or cycling, or an activity you can tolerate. A program that increases aerobic conditioning and strength is optimal. But don't wait until the week before surgery to start; give yourself a minimum of six weeks to get in better shape. A stronger body promotes a better recovery.

Below is a section covering the length of stay, precautions, home safety, and early postoperative exercises for each surgery.

TOTAL KNEE REPLACEMENT

Length of Stay
One to two nights.

Precautions
You will be weight bearing as tolerated (WBAT) on the operated side, unless a complication occurs or preexists, such as a fracture of the tibia, the

shinbone. In such rare cases, the surgeon may write an order for *toe-touch weight bearing* (TTWB) or non-weight bearing (NWB). People who are toe-touch weight bearing are permitted to bear weight on the toes and the ball of the foot of the operated side. And non-weight bearing, to reiterate, means you may not place any weight on the surgical side; this is rarely the case with total knee patients.

The vast majority of total knee patients fall into the first category, weight bearing as tolerated. This means exactly as it sounds. You will be able to put as much weight on the operated side as you can tolerate, and doing so is a good thing. Bearing weight on the prosthesis promotes tissue healing and hastens the return to a normal walking pattern. But you will likely still need an assistive device for a few days to a couple of weeks—the time varies from person to person and depends on other things as well, such as your preexisting state of health, your balance, your pain control, and how far you are walking. You will want to find a smooth and level place to practice walking in the initial stages of recovery. Don't start by walking on grass or gravel, and avoid hills.

A walker is still the device of choice for most knee patients right after surgery. If you have a recent history with crutches and feel comfortable using them, you can definitely do so, but your therapy team will want to see how you walk with them after surgery. Keep in mind that if you are using crutches and one of them catches on a rug as you propel yourself forward, you risk a nasty face plant.

If you are having a minimally invasive knee replacement—a full replacement performed with a less-invasive surgical technique that requires a smaller incision and spares the *quadriceps* muscles around the knee by moving them aside instead of cutting them—you may be able to get by with just a cane, but this depends on your condition and level of alertness after anesthesia. A cane gives you the least amount of support of all the devices, but it does allow you to transfer some of the weight off your surgical leg and into the opposite arm. Most knee patients benefit from having a cane at a later date, after they no longer need a walker, but before they are ready to walk solo. Also, if you are traveling, or walking in unfamiliar territory or for longer distances, it helps to have a cane, especially in the first two months after surgery.

There are no specific movement precautions for total knee patients, although it will feel better if you don't twist your surgical knee. You may bend and straighten it as much as you can, unless instructed otherwise because your incision is not completely closed.

Home Safety

When you go home after your total knee operation, you will spend a lot of time resting, icing your knee, and elevating it above your heart on pillows or a bolster. You will perform the few basic exercises provided here and learn some newer, more difficult ones from your home physical therapist. You will take frequent short walks with your walker, crutches, or cane. Don't try to use this time to build your aerobic capacity or set a new distance record. But don't spend the whole day on the couch, either. Use common sense, and don't overdo it.

If you have stairs at home, you will practice climbing them with a therapist at the hospital before you leave. Here's a quick pre-op primer about stairs.

First, you will need a cane or a crutch *plus* a railing on your stairs. The only exception is if you have one or more platform steps that are deep and wide enough to fit all four feet of a walker. Please do not try to use a walker on regular stairs. This was once taught in the past, but it is now recognized as both unwieldy and unsafe.

Here's why you need a railing: the single most challenging activity for most total knee patients is negotiating a set of stairs. If you don't have a railing and you lose your balance on the stairs, you will fall and likely get hurt. This can also happen if you use two crutches.

When you go up a regular step, you will hold the railing in one hand and the cane or crutch in the other. Hold on to the railing, regardless of whether it is to your left or your right. Then, step up first with the strong leg, followed by the cane and the surgical leg.

When you go down a set of stairs, hold the rail, put your cane down one step, follow with your surgical leg, then your strong leg. One saying therapists use to help patients remember this is, "Up with the good (leg), down with the bad." If you're not already following this sequence at home due to a stiff, painful knee, try practicing it before surgery. It may seem counterintuitive to step down with the surgical leg first, but the upper leg is actually doing the work of lowering your body down with each step; plus the upper leg bends more. You will understand it once you experiment.

Do yourself the favor of investing in a rail on your outdoor or garage stairs, even if there are just a few. If you have stairs at home and can't install one or choose not to, you will need an able-bodied companion to support you. You and your companion will be coached and checked on this in the hospital before being cleared to go home. I have seen many hospital discharges delayed because of patients who could not master the stairs.

Other home-safety advice: some people benefit from having a raised toilet seat, a bedside commode, especially if the sleeping quarters are not close to a bathroom, and a chair to sit on in the shower or tub (you won't be allowed to take a bath until the incision is completely healed, to prevent infection). A hand-held showerhead is also recommended if you sit down. A reacher is another handy tool for picking things up from the floor without bending down, but it is not essential if you have help at home. You will have a chance to discuss these devices with your occupational therapist in the hospital. These adaptive devices are typically not covered by insurance, except workers' compensation.

Exercises

The purpose of early exercise is twofold. Moving the surgical leg as well as the body in general is part of a multifaceted strategy to prevent blood clots from forming. Depending on your medication history, you will also be given a blood thinner to help in this regard. The second reason to begin exercises as soon as possible is to gain early mobility in the new knee and to proactively combat stiffness.

The knee is a hinge joint that moves primarily in two directions, *flexion*, or bending, and *extension*, or straightening. It will feel swollen and painful after surgery and also somewhat numb in patches on the skin. It may hurt when you first move it, but then it will feel a little better. If you don't move it at all for a day or so, it will be much more difficult to overcome that tight, stiff, swollen feeling. Some stiffness is inevitable, but regularly moving your knee will help tremendously.

The easiest exercise, called an ankle pump, simply involves pointing and flexing your entire foot so that you feel your calf muscles contracting. You will do this while lying in your hospital bed. This exercise also helps to prevent blood clots.

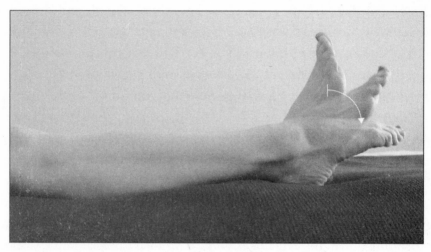

Photograph by Travis Tucker; model is Nancy Orr.

Other exercises you will learn while lying down include quad sets, glut sets, and heel slides. Quad sets involve tightening the quadriceps muscles—the muscles around the knee that are responsible for straightening it. The quads contract (or tighten) when you push the thigh downward. Quad sets

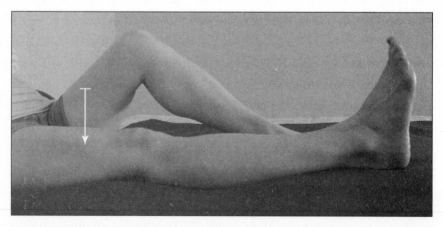

Photograph by Travis Tucker; model is Nancy Orr.

are the easiest in a series of progressive exercises for regaining the strength in these crucial muscles, which are now weaker on the surgical side.

Glut sets are simply contracting the buttocks muscles. You can do them sitting, standing, or lying down. While these are especially important for total hip patients, some knee patients with chronic pain who have favored their surgical leg for months or years also have atrophied gluteal muscles on that side. Whenever possible, physical therapists also try to address the muscle groups in the joints above and below the surgery—in this case, the hip and the ankle.

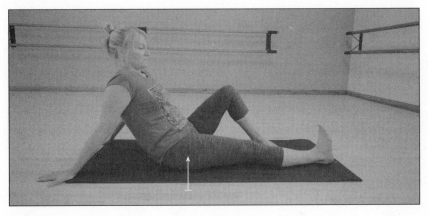

Photograph by Travis Tucker; model is Nancy Orr.

Heel slides are your first active attempt to bend or flex your knee, and these entail sliding your heel toward your buttock on the surgical side while lying on your back or propping yourself up on your elbows. These are the

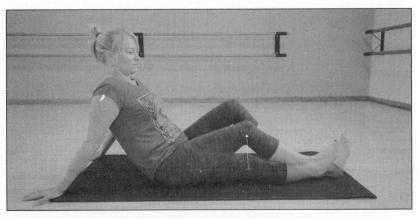

Photograph by Travis Tucker; model is Nancy Orr.

most difficult of the first four exercises, but you will notice how much more you can move after you get started, as they reduce stiffness.

You may have difficulty straightening your knee completely after surgery. It is possible you have tight *hamstrings*, the muscles on the back of the thigh that bend the knee. Your physical therapist may place a small rolled-up towel under your Achilles tendon when you are lying on your back and ask you to leave it there for a period of time, such as ten minutes. This gravity-assisted activity will encourage your knee to straighten or extend more fully, and you may need to repeat it several times daily. Also, it is best to avoid sleeping with a pillow under your knee, as this encourages the hamstrings to tighten up again.

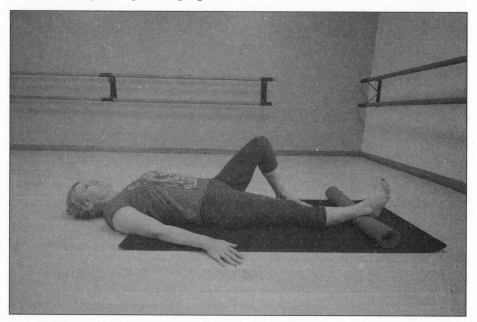

Photograph by Travis Tucker; model is Nancy Orr.

More advanced exercises may be initiated in the hospital or at home with your visiting therapist. They include two exercises performed while lying flat or partially upright, the short-arc quad and the straight-leg raise, and two others performed in a seated position, called seated knee flexion and seated knee extension.

The short-arc quad is a more difficult exercise for strengthening the quadriceps than a quad set because it involves straightening the knee against the added effect of gravity.

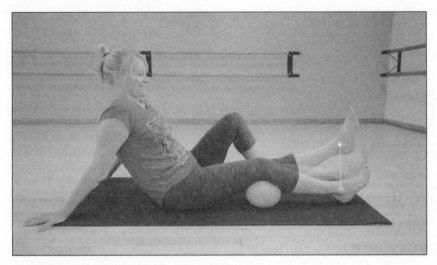

Photograph by Travis Tucker; model is Nancy Orr.

The straight-leg raise requires that you keep your knee straight while lifting the whole thigh. Lie down with your operated leg straight and your other knee bent to protect your back. Slowly lift the surgical leg up in the air to the level of the opposite knee, then slowly lower it back down.

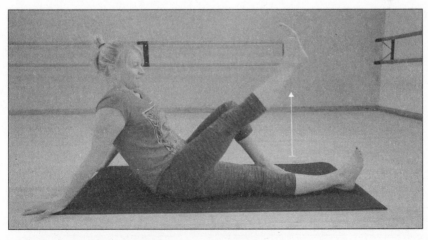

Photograph by Travis Tucker; model is Nancy Orr.

Seated exercises are also great for your knees. To work on bending, sit in a straight-backed chair with your feet on the floor. Slide the foot of the surgical leg back as far as you can under the chair, using the opposite foot if necessary to bend it farther.

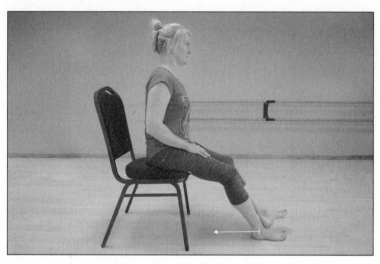

Photograph by Travis Tucker; model is Nancy Orr.

To work on extension, sit in the chair, both feet on the floor. Keeping your back upright, try to straighten the surgical leg. You may use your other foot to help; this will challenge your core muscles, but try not to slouch.

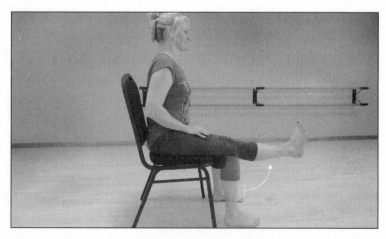

Photograph by Travis Tucker; model is Nancy Orr.

As you progress with physical therapy, you will continue to work on flexion and extension, and on strengthening all of your thigh and lower leg muscles. Over time, you should be able to regain flexion that is nearly equal to that in your other knee (between 120 and 140 degrees), as well as complete extension (0 degrees), both of which can be measured by a physical therapist with a tool called a *goniometer*, a device that looks like a protractor.

TOTAL HIP REPLACEMENT

Length of Stay
One to two nights.

Precautions
For traditional (posterior or lateral) total hip replacement: For the first six weeks after surgery, no flexing the hip past 90 degrees, which means no lifting the knee higher than the hip, or bending your upper body forward past a position that is parallel to the floor when standing; no crossing the surgical leg over the midline of your body; no turning the surgical leg inward, as in a pigeon-toed position. Avoiding these movements, especially the latter two at the same time, protects the hip from possible dislocation.

For anterior total hip replacement: For the first six weeks, no extending the surgical leg backward and outward at the same time; avoid extreme movements in any direction, such as bending over to touch the floor. Some surgeons who perform the anterior approach do not order any precautions.

Most total hip patients, regardless of the surgical technique used, will be weight bearing as tolerated (WBAT) and will begin walking with a front-wheeled walker or crutches on level surfaces, and will use a cane on stairs.

Home Safety
Remove loose rugs and obstacles from the floor, and make sure pets aren't so rambunctious as to knock you over.

If you have traditional hip precautions, you will need to sit in chairs that are high enough to allow your knee to remain below the level of your hip. For the same reason, you may need a raised toilet seat; one thing you can do ahead of surgery is measure the height of your toilet and share this information with your occupational therapist at the hospital. He or she can then assess whether you need a raised toilet seat.

Another specialty item for patients with traditional hip precautions is a hip kit, which consists of a reacher for picking up things and pulling up your pants, a sock aid for putting on your socks without help, and a long-handled sponge for bathing your lower body. Some hip kits also include a long-handled shoehorn for help sliding your feet into your shoes. A hip kit may be purchased in advance at a medical supply store, online, or at the hospital. If you have anterior hip precautions, you may not need a hip kit.

If the entrance to your home includes one or more platform steps that are deep and wide enough to accommodate all four legs of your walker, you may negotiate them without a railing, but you should have a companion by your side the first few times. Get as close as possible to the first step and lift the walker up and onto the platform. (If you are too far away from the step, lifting the walker with outstretched arms could throw you forward and off balance.) Step up first with your strong leg, then bring up the surgical leg. Repeat the process for other platform steps and also use this technique when ascending a curb from the street to the sidewalk. When descending, lower the walker first, followed by the surgical leg, then the strong leg.

For regular indoor or outdoor stairs, you will need a railing and a cane or a crutch. Hold the railing, and carry the cane in the opposite hand. Step up first with the strong leg, and follow with the operated leg, pushing on the cane and pulling on the railing as needed.

To descend, hold the rail and the cane in opposite hands. Place the cane down first, then the surgical leg, followed by the good leg. Think of the mantra, "up with the good, down with the bad," meaning that you always lead with the strong leg when ascending and with the weaker, surgical leg when descending.

Exercises

The introductory exercises for total hip patients are the same as those for total knee patients, and include ankle pumps, quad sets, glut sets, and heel slides, which are illustrated above. In addition, you may be taught at least one exercise to strengthen your *hip abductors*, the muscles that move your leg out to the side. These muscles are very important for balance; they are typically weak in total hip patients, as well as in the population in general.

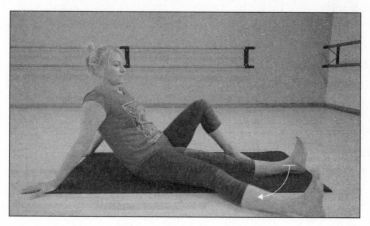

Photograph by Travis Tucker; model is Nancy Orr.

If you do this lying down, it is easier with a non-sticky surface underneath the thigh, such as a silky sheet or a plastic bag, so that your leg slides out to the side without getting stuck. You may also try it in a standing position; just be sure to hold on to something solid for balance.

There is a new trend among some orthopedic surgeons of not ordering any physical therapy for total hip patients after discharge from the hospital.[10] In the past, most total hip patients had home physical therapy for a week or two, followed by outpatient therapy; now, most do not receive home therapy, and some do not receive outpatient therapy. This is particularly true for anterior hip patients, for whom the reinforcement of precautions is not crucial to prevent dislocation.

As a physical therapist, I take issue with this new development. Here's why: How would you know what to do, how much of it to do, and how often to do it? How would you know how to strengthen your hip muscles, regain optimal balance, and progress the rehabilitation program correctly and safely on your own, without any monitoring?

Walking is not enough after a total hip replacement. A home exercise program given in the hospital may include a few standing exercises. But are you doing them correctly? And after you have mastered them, will you know what to do next? Do you know what exercises and movements are better avoided? How would you? And if you wish to return to sports, such as tennis, or skiing or other activities that require rapid and repetitive side-to-side movement and good balance, physical therapy can make a big difference in both safety and skill.

Additionally, if you have been sidelined for a long time with hip pain and have become overweight in the process, physical therapy will help you target weakened muscles while also supporting a safe weight-loss program.

You may only need a few sessions of outpatient physical therapy, and they can be spread out. My advice is to talk to your doctor ahead of surgery about it, and remind him of goals you have to return to specific activities. While hip surgeons may not automatically prescribe outpatient physical therapy, most are willing to do so when asked.

TOTAL SHOULDER REPLACEMENT

Length of Stay
One to two nights.

Precautions for Traditional Total Shoulder Replacement
First, do not bear weight on the surgical-side arm for six weeks, which means no pushing up with that arm from a bed or chair. Second, no *external rotation*—if you stand with arms at your side and bend your elbows, with your thumbs pointing to the ceiling, external rotation would consist of moving your forearm outward, away from your body. This motion puts stress on the surgical site.

The third precaution is that you may not lift the arm at the shoulder joint, as if you were reaching for something on a high shelf or hailing a cab. This movement is called *shoulder flexion*. You may bend your arm at the elbow joint, but do not try to lift the whole arm up in the air. Instead, as an exercise, you may be shown how to use the opposite hand to lift the surgical arm. You will likely be given a sling or shoulder brace to wear for a period of time. The directions vary as to when you may remove it, so it is advisable to ask your surgeon for some basic guidelines in advance.

Precautions for a Reverse Total Shoulder Replacement

This is a newer surgery, pioneered in the United States by orthopedic surgeon Paul Grammont in the mid-eighties and approved by the Food and Drug Administration in 2004, for people with end-stage arthritis who no longer have functioning rotator cuff muscles.[11]

To expand on the description of a reverse total shoulder replacement given earlier in the chapter, first consider the normal shoulder. The high end of the arm bone, or humeral head, has the convex shape of a ball. The site where it attaches to the scapula, or shoulder blade, is called the glenoid cavity; it resembles a saucer.

Now, imagine that the humeral head is flattened into a saucer shape, and the cavity in the shoulder blade turns into a ball. Each surface becomes its opposite. This is a reverse total shoulder. The reverse total shoulder allows for the deltoid muscles to compensate for the impaired rotator cuff complex, meaning you can lift and rotate the arm again, but without arthritic pain. You will regain some though not all normal shoulder mobility after a reverse total shoulder, but the motion should be pain-free.

While precautions for the reverse total shoulder replacement vary by surgeon and by individual patient, they typically include no weight bearing (NWB) on the surgical arm for six weeks, plus some variation of no moving the elbow backward, no lifting the arm out to the side (like a chicken wing), and no twisting your arm to reach your low back.

Home Safety

You may not need any new adaptive equipment after a total shoulder operation except perhaps a reacher, which you could use with your strong side to retrieve things from a closet or the floor. However, you will need hands-on help in the initial days and weeks with dressing and showering. You will be able to write and to use eating utensils with your surgical-side hand, but you may not be able to brush your teeth, comb your hair, or tend to personal hygiene (wiping). Think about these temporary disabilities in advance, and if surgery is on your dominant side, practice doing these tasks with your nondominant arm and hand.

Exercises

You will be encouraged to open and close your fist and to flex (bend) and extend your wrist. You will be allowed to bend and straighten your elbow—think *biceps* curl—without moving your shoulder.

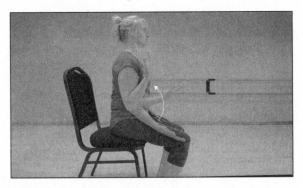

Photograph by Travis Tucker; model is Nancy Orr.

For both types of shoulder replacements, your hospital physical or occupational therapist may teach an odd-looking exercise called a pendulum, which is a gravity-assisted movement of the new joint that gives it a safe and gentle stretch.

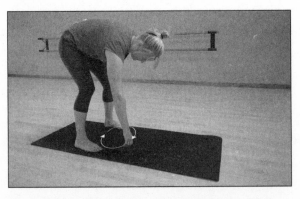

Photograph by Travis Tucker; model is Nancy Orr.

Your surgeon will prescribe outpatient therapy several weeks after the operation so that you keep gaining movement and strength in your arm.

SPINE FUSION SURGERY

Length of Stay

One to four days, depending on how many vertebrae are fused and the operative approach used by the surgeon.

Precautions

For both lumbar and cervical spine fusion: no bending forward from the surgical region, no lifting more than five to ten pounds (a gallon of milk weighs eight pounds), and no twisting the spine at the surgical area. In other words, no bending, lifting, or twisting, a.k.a. NO BLT. Your movement may initially resemble a robot's.

Also, after a cervical fusion, you shouldn't raise your arms overhead. You may be fitted with a hard-plastic brace, such as a Miami J collar, to wear all of the time except when you shower. For showering, you may receive a different brace, such as an Aspen collar. By preventing the prohibited movements, these braces help to promote the union (fusion) of the vertebral bones.

If you are having a low-back fusion, you may be fitted with a neoprene brace with metal stays. This type of brace provides compression, which may feel supportive, but it is less rigid than a plastic brace. It discourages but won't absolutely prevent the prohibited movements. If your surgery involves an anterior approach—through the belly—you most likely won't need a brace, nor would one feel comfortable in the front.

The trickiest challenge for most low-back patients is learning how to get in and out of bed correctly, by using a maneuver called the log roll. You will learn and practice the log roll in the hospital, but you will do yourself a favor by learning it on your own and practicing it ahead of surgery. Some back patients are already well versed with the log roll when they come in, having figured it out on their own.

Let's start with your sleeping position. You will be encouraged to sleep on your side with knees bent, or on your back with a bolster under your knees. If you are on your back, the bolster should be removed when you get up. With bent knees, practice rolling to one side and to the other, and decide which side is easiest for you to get out of your bed at home. You want to roll so that your lower legs can drop over the edge of the bed. As they do, bring yourself up to a seated position by pushing up with the upper hand (the one farthest from the bed). Push with this hand and then let go, because if you leave it planted on the bed, you will twist.

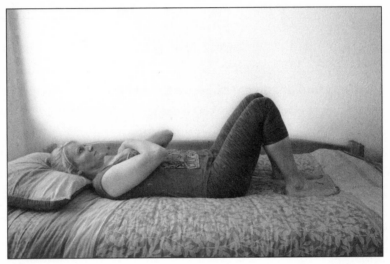

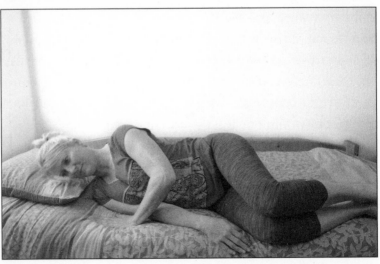

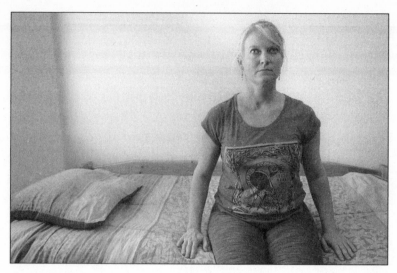

Photographs by Travis Tucker; model is Nancy Orr.

To get back into bed, sit down on the edge first, with a straight back, and move your hips toward the center of the bed as one unit, without shimmying one side and then the other. If your bed is high, you may benefit from a small step on the side, but be careful not to trip on it. Once you are sitting, let your forearm and head drop toward the pillow in one smooth motion, without twisting, and also bring your feet up onto the bed. From this side-lying position, you can roll onto your back. If you need to shift around in bed, try not to lift up your hips or shimmy; go to a side-lying position first, then slide your hips very slowly and carefully to reposition, or ask for help from someone who can pull very gently on the sheet beneath you.

Home Safety

A front-wheeled walker is helpful, especially if you have leg weakness prior to surgery, or if you are unsteady for any reason. A walker gives you support and stability and allows you to walk a longer distance early on in the healing process. You will probably just push it like a shopping cart.

If you are a cervical patient, you probably won't need a walking device, unless you already use one. When you turn, you will need to move like a robot, turning your whole body at once, without twisting. Take extra care on stairs, because you need to look straight ahead, not down. Try counting the number of stairs ahead of time, then count each one out loud as you go up and come down. This technique will let you know when to expect to land on the top step as well as the bottom one. Be sure to have a solid railing along your stairs.

Plan to sit in a straight-backed chair with armrests at home—armrests let you push up with your hands. Recliners, or other soft-backed chairs or couches that enable slouching, are discouraged. It's okay to have someone put pillows behind your back when you sit. In the hospital, we often put pillows vertically behind the back to provide a comfortable leaning surface, but the back should remain straight.

A spine kit may come in handy. This is similar to a hip kit—with a reacher, long-handled sponge, a sock aid, and possibly a long-handled shoe-horn. Your occupational therapist may also discuss toilet tongs. Depending on your size and anatomy, you may need them to perform personal hygiene without twisting your back. Other equipment to consider and to discuss with the hospital occupational therapist is a tub bench, a hand-held showerhead, and a raised toilet seat. You may not need all of these things, depending on your home setup and your presurgical condition.

Exercises

There are no early exercises for post-op spine patients, because it is too soon to move the spine or strengthen the core muscles around it. It is okay to perform ankle pumps and quad sets while lying in bed (see illustrations above), but the best thing you can do is walk. Walking, because it is a weight-bearing activity, is believed to stimulate bone growth. Some surgeons expect patients to be able to walk two miles by their first follow-up visit, usually in ten days, although this may seem like too much. If the weather is cold or wet, find a mall; take your walker and a companion and walk every day. Your hospital therapist can advise you on starting an individualized and realistic walking program.

In addition to teaching you the log roll, physical and occupational therapists will show you how to stand up and sit down correctly—hint: with a straight back—and how to perform everyday tasks safely, such as brushing your teeth—hint: it's better to drool into a cup than to lean over. You will also practice going up and down stairs. Once you demonstrate that you can move safely and follow your precautions, you may be discharged by the therapy staff, meaning that the physical and occupational therapists have cleared you to go home. This could happen a day or more before you are actually discharged from the hospital. The therapy team should advise you and your providers that you still need to get up and walk, but now you can do it with a family member, your nurse, or nursing assistant. You will still need to alert your nurse first, to make sure your vital signs are stable and your lines are correctly detached.

TOTAL ANKLE REPLACEMENT

Length of Stay
One to two nights.

Precautions
You will be non-weight bearing (NWB), meaning you may not put any weight on the surgical foot. This will be your greatest challenge for about six weeks. The non-weight bearing rule can come as a rude awakening. I have seen many post-op ankle patients who had no idea they would be non-weight bearing. Either their surgeon didn't tell them or the meaning of this rule didn't sink in. These patients were consequently ill prepared to return home. Their inability to comply with the non-weight bearing status meant that they were confined to a wheelchair or a knee scooter. Many ended up recovering in a skilled nursing facility.

After surgery, your ankle will be immobilized by a splint placed on the back of the calf, and this will be held in place by a large bulky dressing wrapped around the lower leg. Later, once the swelling has subsided, you will likely be fitted with a knee-high boot to protect the ankle while it continues to heal. The result is that your foot will feel heavy.

If you wish to recover at home versus at a skilled nursing facility, I would highly recommend that you learn how to use crutches or a walker before surgery. Practice using them at home without putting any weight on the surgical foot.

If you can't hop safely in a walker or crutches, even from the bedroom to the bathroom at home, then a hospital therapist may be able to teach a family member how to help you transfer from a wheelchair to a chair, a bed, and a toilet. But the family member will need to be with you most of the time, if not 24/7. Consider, if you were alone, how you would get out of your home in the event of a fire or other emergency.

You will not be able to use a walker, scooter, or wheelchair on stairs. If you have stairs at home that you must negotiate, practice ahead of time with one crutch and a rail. Hold the railing in one hand and push down on the crutch's hand piece with the other. If possible, hold the second crutch in the same hand, or try holding it perpendicular to the first one. Try hopping up, one step at a time, on your strong foot. This is less difficult if you have good upper body strength. Going upstairs with one crutch in each hand is less safe because you aren't holding on to something fixed, and if one crutch slips, you will almost certainly lose your balance. A cane (even with a railing) does not provide adequate support if you are non-weight bearing.

To come down the stairs, hold both crutches in one hand if possible (opposite the railing) or slide one crutch all the way down so it will be waiting when you get there. Lower the crutch first, then lower your surgical foot part way without putting weight on it, then gently lower the good foot. Coming down is easier than climbing up.

If you can't manage the stairs with a crutch and a rail, ask your hospital therapist about bumping. This means sitting on a stair, facing downwards, and using your arms and your nonsurgical foot to lift your hips and body up, one step at a time, going backward. It's surprisingly easy to master, but it is a time-consuming task, and you will tire of it. Plus, you will need to stand up at the top and get back to your device, whether crutches, walker, wheelchair, or scooter. The same is true for when you go downstairs.

If all of this seems overwhelming or too difficult, you are not alone. A skilled nursing facility is sometimes the best and safest option, because you will get daily therapy there and learn which devices work best for you.

There, for instance, you may learn how to use a sliding board (a plastic or wooden board that serves as a bridge to your destination). One end of the board goes under one buttock as you sit in a wheelchair (the wheelchair must have removable armrests and locked brakes), and the other end goes on top of your target surface, such as the bed. Once the sliding board is securely in place, you will use your arms and upper body to slide on your buttocks from the wheelchair to the bed.

Another option is to ask your surgeon to prescribe a few outpatient physical therapy sessions in advance of surgery so that you can try to master some or all of these tasks ahead of time. Many states no longer require a prescription for physical therapy, but check with your insurance plan for details about what is covered.[12] If your surgeon doesn't write an order, consider asking your primary care physician.

Home Safety

Once you resolve the walking conundrum, other issues should be easier. You may need a bath bench for sitting in the shower or the tub. You should remove all small rugs in areas where you will be walking. Measure the width of your bathroom door to be sure your assistive device will fit through. A reacher may come in handy so you don't have to pick up things from the floor.

Exercises

Since your ankle will be immobilized by the splint, you will not be given exercises in the hospital except to wiggle your toes, which promotes circulation and also fights stiffness. Your therapists in the hospital will work with you on getting out of bed, transferring to a chair and a toilet, and walking a short distance in a walker or crutches, such as to the bathroom. When you are not icing the lower leg and elevating it above the level of the heart, you may sit and practice straightening each knee from a bent position, to build thigh strength. Armchair pushups are good for building upper-body strength, and they can be done ahead of time. Simply sit in a chair with armrests, put your surgical leg in front of you and out of the way, and push up with your arms and the good leg. Build up to two sets of fifteen repetitions. This will increase strength in the back muscles (the *latissimus dorsi*) that you need to use crutches or a walker as well as the *triceps* muscles on the back of the arm. To strengthen the nonoperative leg and prepare it for doing more work, try three daily sets of ten to fifteen one-legged squats. Place one hand against a wall or on the back of a chair to maintain your balance.

Chapter 3

You Can't Go Home Alone

The first two weeks after a major orthopedic surgery aren't exactly a picnic, unless your picnic includes fire ants and three-legged races in the living room. Just because you are discharged home one or two days after surgery doesn't mean you are ready to take care of yourself. For a few days, at least, you will need much of the same type of care you received in the hospital, including meal prep and delivery, help with finding a comfortable position and changing your ice, and assistance in keeping track of your medications. You and your caregiver should keep a written log of your medication times and dosages. You should have someone there at night, when falls are most likely to occur.

Expect to have someone standing by when you take your first few showers and when you walk up and down stairs. If all of this sounds frightening, it doesn't need to be. It is completely normal to feel weak, tired, and in some degree of pain. The body's natural response to an invasion like surgery is to send its army of tiny immune soldiers marching into the battlefield of healing. This is where your energy is going. If you try to go it alone you are taking unnecessary risks.

A BAD MEMORY

I once had a knee-replacement patient, Donny, who was in his midseventies and lived alone. He was an athletic man and still looked fit and wiry.

But Donny had a memory problem. After my third *and* fourth sessions working with him, Donny asked, "Have I met you before?" He had also asked this at the second and third sessions. I apparently hadn't left much of an impression.

The nurse assigned to Donny on the scheduled day of discharge, a Saturday, attributed his forgetfulness to the side effects of the pain medications. This was a reasonable assumption. But I had watched Donny for two days, and I suspected there was something grimmer behind his cognitive status. He was alert, but he was losing large chunks of time. He would learn a new task and execute it, then completely forget it the next time I saw him. One night he got out of bed alone, despite repeated instructions from staff and signs saying, "Call, don't fall." The night staff installed a bed alarm so they would be alerted if he tried to do it again. I was very concerned about Donny's safety, yet he wanted to go home by himself.

Donny was widowed, had a son in another city, and said he didn't have anybody to stay with him. He insisted he would be fine alone at home, but after the occupational therapist, the case manager, and I all talked to him about our concerns, he finally agreed to go to a skilled nursing facility until he regained his independence, and hopefully, his judgment. Like many patients, Donny did not have a regular primary care physician. His preoperative physical was done at the hospital, and we lacked knowledge of his prior cognitive capacity, such as whether he had been diagnosed with early dementia.

On that Saturday morning when Donny was to discharge to the skilled nursing facility, I had one final session with him. His nurse, Scott, who only worked Saturdays, said Donny was doing well and seemed mentally clear. In fact, Scott said, Donny had backed out of the agreement, made just the day before, to go to the skilled nursing facility. A man and woman were visiting him in his room; they said they were friends of Donny's and they would take him home and stay with him 24/7 for a few days. None of this rang true to me, and as the person who had spent the most time with Donny, I disagreed with the plan. But Donny had convinced the Saturday hospitalist, the medical doctor filling in for the regular hospitalist (see chapter 5), the rounding surgeon (not his own surgeon, but a partner who didn't know Donny), and Scott that he was fine to go home. And so, in spite of my concerns, which I communicated to all parties and documented in my notes, the friends took him home.

That was the last I heard about Donny until two Saturdays later, when Scott came up to me, and said, "Liz, you remember that guy, Donny? Well, you were absolutely right about him, and I was wrong."

The same evening he had left, Donny called the hospital in a panic. He couldn't find his pain meds. The prescription had been written and documented in the chart, and the couple had promised to take him to fill it. Donny could not remember whether the script had been filled and if so, where the pills were. He had searched everywhere, he said. Donny pleaded with Scott to let him come back and "get more pills." This was not an option, legally, and Scott had told Donny he would need to get in touch with the orthopedic office. There was no mention of the friends.

I suspected Donny had simply summoned the friends to show up at the hospital and state that they were staying with him. When he called Scott, the friends were no longer available.

"I don't know what he ended up doing," Scott told me.

Donny's example is unfortunate, but patients do have responsibilities, and their actions are sometimes not in their own best interests.

My theory was that Donny had some underlying dementia that he was hiding, and the narcotics added to his confusion. It's also possible he was seeking more drugs because of a prior habit. Either way, as someone who had lived alone for a long time, he was stubbornly independent and didn't want to accept help. Maybe he feared that he would never leave the nursing home. This is a common concern among older people whose health is compromised or who are frail. But even though there may be permanent residents housed in a skilled nursing facility, they are almost always part of a different population than those who are rehabilitating from a joint replacement. Joint and spine patients receive at least one hour of daily therapy in a skilled nursing facility, and once they make enough progress to take care of themselves, they go home. In the meantime, they get the vital help they need.

THE NEED FOR COMPASSIONATE CARE

Even if you are completely sound of mind, you will still need support at home. During the first few days after your surgery, you will probably function at a much-reduced capacity—survival mode. You are a bit like a sick child who needs tending.

Narcotics make most people not just sleepy but constipated, so you will need to take stool softeners and drink more water than usual. They also make many people nauseous; other medications will address that problem. Don't stay in bed, unless instructed to do so, but know that getting showered and dressed will zap your energy for the morning, and you will soon want to retreat to the couch. You may not be able to stay awake long enough to watch a movie, much less read a book. Forget about cleaning up, or doing any chores. Meaningful work is out of the question for most people. The only thing motivating you to leave the couch, or the chair if you are a spine patient, is the need to use the bathroom, or, if you are a knee patient, to greet your home therapist at the door.

Fortunately, the first few days are so forgettable that you will hopefully forget them. Not your caregiver. It can be a challenge. The caregiver works like a Sherpa to carry your things, bring you food, water, ice, and medication, take you to the bathroom, and help position you comfortably with just the right pillows in all the right places. This personal attendant will have little time to care for his or her own needs, much less tackle the household chores. And if you have just one caregiver, the emotional support and reassurance also falls to this person. He or she may be counting on you to return the favor at a later date. Husbands and wives often say this: "I did it for her/him. Now it's my turn."

Orthopedic surgeon Ira Kirschenbaum, MD, chronicled his own experience with a total knee replacement in www.medscape.com.[13]

"I don't believe that anyone can go through a knee replacement operation alone," he wrote. "You either need a mobile and dedicated caregiver twenty-four hours a day for a solid two weeks or you need to go to some type of rehab hospital." Further, he added, "patients who live alone or have limited caregivers at home cannot go home immediately after surgery."

Of course, not everybody has a spouse, a partner, or a child who can help. So what are your options if you live alone?

If you have a close friend, you can ask the friend to stay with you for a few nights and find other friends to come and check on you during the day. Or, you can see about staying at a close friend's home, if that is easier. You can offer to compensate the friends later with an in-kind gesture.

Second, you can hire someone to come and help you at home. There are many home-care companies, such as Home Instead, Visiting Angels, or Comfort Care, that provide trained caregivers (as opposed to medical professionals) at an hourly wage. One drawback for this option is that it will not be covered by health insurance.

Why then, you may ask, can't I just go to a skilled nursing facility for a week or two until I'm strong enough to be alone at home? That's not how the system works. If you sail through the hospital experience and meet all of your therapy goals, as many people do, you do not need skilled inpatient care. Donny needed skilled care because he demonstrated poor judgment, moved unsafely, and lacked the understanding to manage his own medications. Maybe you need home physical therapy, but if you do really well, you don't need the level of care provided in a skilled nursing facility, and insurance may not cover it.

Your choice of discharge destination is something important to discuss with your surgeon ahead of time. Many, if not most, surgeons today prefer that their patients go directly home rather than to a rehab center. As the mobility and safety experts, therapists also weigh in on this decision when working with you postoperatively. If a patient continues to move unsafely after several therapy sessions, the physical and occupational therapists will recommend skilled care upon discharge. The patient can refuse a professional's recommendation, like Donny did, but the aim is to reach a consensus.

Insurance covers skilled care, but it does not cover unskilled care. Skilled care means the professional care of a doctor, nurse, a physical or occupational therapist, or a nursing assistant. For instance, if you have a complex medical condition that requires a regular adjustment of medications, or if you were independent before and are now unable to get out of bed, walk, or negotiate stairs on your own, you may qualify for a skilled nursing facility. You must require the skilled services of a nurse, such as a daily blood draw, or close heart monitoring, or regular wound care, to name a few examples, and you will also receive daily physical therapy and perhaps occupational therapy as an extension of what you started in the hospital.

If you are medically stable and able to go home, you can receive physical and occupational therapy there, which is covered by insurance, but each therapist comes only a couple of times per week, depending on your diagnosis. The home therapist teaches you how to progress specific skills, such as strengthening your knee or negotiating stairs. But there are limits: a physical therapist is not there to prepare meals, or to pick up your medications or groceries at the store.

That is the realm of "unskilled" care, which is defined as routine tasks that do not require the expertise of a professional: preparing and serving meals, cleaning, doing laundry, getting ice, running errands, and providing companionship. These make up the caregiver's job.

The take-home message: invest your time ahead of surgery in lining up a reliable support team for the first few days or a week after surgery. This can pose a greater challenge if you live alone, but you can do it! You and your home caregiver will determine fairly quickly how much help you need, for how many days, and when it is safe for you to be alone for a few hours. You will be grateful for the help.

Chapter 4

Know Your Lines

This chapter isn't about memorizing a script or even having your questions lined up for the surgeon, although that is advised. The lines identified here are your lifelines—all the equipment attached to you when you wake up from surgery. You will become aware of some of them in the recovery suite, and the rest in your room. You may not be able to move much. Parts of your body will feel heavy, weighed down, or numb. Try to relax. It is only temporary. Sensations will return soon enough.

LINES FOR EVERYONE

Starting at the head and ending at the toes, what follows is a description of the common tubes and devices you are likely to encounter no matter which orthopedic surgery you are having. After this section, look under your specific topic for even more items.

Nasal Cannula

The cannula is the clear, forked tube delivering oxygen that is draped over your ears and fits in your nostrils. You were given supplemental oxygen while under anesthesia, and you will continue to need extra oxygen for a period of time.

You may decide that you don't like or need this tube in your nose and remove it. An alarm will sound, and your nurse or another clinician will come in, put it back on, and ask that you please leave it there.

Oxygen levels are important right now—and they are being monitored to make sure you are getting enough, but not more than you need. A temporary reduction in your oxygen intake won't do any harm, but if your numbers are low for long periods of time, you won't feel well and your recovery may be compromised. The condition of having low oxygen in your blood is called *hypoxemia*.

All of your vital organs and tissues are perfused by the oxygen that is carried on the hemoglobin molecules in your blood. When your organs and tissues do not get enough oxygen, the surgical wound does not heal as well. During surgery, anesthesia inhibits your oxygen intake; after surgery, narcotics inhibit it again. When your breathing is shallow, your lungs are temporarily more susceptible to fluid buildup.

Oxygen volume is measured in liters per minute; a typical level for a healthy person to receive after surgery is two liters per minute. You may need oxygen during your first night after surgery, but over time, you should need less. If you can see your own monitor, the number followed by a percent sign is your oxygen saturation, a measure of oxygen absorbed by the hemoglobin in your blood. A healthy number is 88 percent or above, but this can vary depending on your medical condition. If your levels drop below an amount the nurse has programmed into the monitor, an alarm will sound.

There are two things you can do to speed up the process of saying goodbye to the tube in your nose: practice taking slow, deep breaths, and be diligent about using your incentive spirometer if you are given one.

The incentive spirometer is a plastic device with a tube and a mouthpiece attached. As you breathe in deeply through the mouthpiece, a cylinder moves upward to measure the volume of air you are inhaling. Your nurse will give you a target milliliter level and instruct you to use the device ten times per hour, more or less. Deep breathing with the incentive spirometer exercises your lungs and helps to prevent mucus buildup that could lead to pneumonia.

If your oxygen levels are on the low side when you leave the hospital, you may be sent home with a portable tank of oxygen, and an appointment with a service provider to deliver a larger tank to your home and set you up with a prescribed amount. Don't be discouraged by this. It should be a temporary inconvenience if you did not use oxygen prior to surgery.

If you have sleep apnea and use a continuous positive airway pressure (CPAP) machine at night, ask a contact person in your surgeon's office if you should bring your own mask and machine to the hospital.

Pulse Oximeter

The pulse oximeter, or pulse ox, is a small, clothespin-like device that commonly attaches around a fingertip and reads your oxygen saturation. Again, the target should be 88 percent or higher. On occasion, patients find the pulse ox on a toe or perhaps an ear, where it is attached with a special sensor. A long cord stretches from the pulse ox to your monitor, where your heart rate and oxygen saturation are brightly displayed. If you are asked to remove nail polish from your fingers and toes before surgery, the reason is that polish and other coatings such as acrylic can interfere with the conductivity of the pulse ox.

How, you may wonder, does a little device on your finger read your oxygen saturation? Very simply, it sends a red light into your hemoglobin cells in the blood and measures the percentage of light that is absorbed by the hemoglobin cells (versus the light coming out the other side). The higher the absorption of red light by the hemoglobin cells, the higher the oxygen saturation.

A normal heart rate at rest for most people ranges from 55 to 80 beats per minute. When you walk outside your room, your therapist can detach your pulse-ox line from the monitor and substitute it with a handheld monitor to see how your oxygen saturation and heart rate respond to increased activity.

Intravenous (IV) Lines

You may have an intravenous (IV) line in each arm or hand, depending on where suitable veins were found. Why do you need two of them, you may ask? One IV may be used to deliver fluids such as a saline solution to maintain hydration and deliver medication, while the other is a backup in case the first one becomes infiltrated, or clogged. If you need a blood transfusion, one IV will be needed for several hours to deliver it. One misconception people have is that there are needles in their arms—there aren't.

The needle was withdrawn after the tubing went in, and the tube is tiny and flexible. If your IV becomes infiltrated, or if it becomes loose, you may see blood coming out of the site. There's no need to panic, but let your nurse know because the line is no longer functioning.

The IV bags will hang on a pole on either side of your bed.

Round Sticky Pads

If you find round things sticking to your back, chest, or elsewhere, you may peel them off. These were attachment sites for electrocardiogram (ECG) leads to monitor your heart rate and rhythm during surgery. It is possible you will have another ECG during the hospital stay, a painless procedure, but new pads will be attached.

Blood Pressure Cuff

When you arrive in your room after surgery, a blood pressure cuff will be wrapped around one arm, just above the elbow. It may be set on an automatic inflating timer, as frequently as every thirty minutes at first, and the squeezing sensation can be annoying. Blood pressure also shows up on your monitor as the systolic pressure on top—this number is the maximum pressure in your arteries when the heart beats—and the diastolic pressure on the bottom—the maximum arterial pressure between beats when the heart is filling with oxygenated blood. If your blood pressure is too low, for instance if your systolic pressure drops below 80 when it is normally 120, you may feel lightheaded or nauseous, and you may be given extra fluids in your IV line to increase your pressure.

If your baseline blood pressure runs high and you normally take medication, your doctors may reduce the dosage during the hospital stay, while carefully monitoring your pressure. It is more typical for blood pressure to drop than to increase in the hours after surgery.

Foley Catheter

You may view your Foley catheter as a blessing or a curse. This is the tube that collects your urine and stores it in a clear bag hooked to the side of the bed. The Foley will be inserted by a nurse or doctor in the operating room

when you are asleep. The catheter bag collects urine when you are uncon-
scious and unable to control your bladder. It also allows for measurement
of your fluid output after surgery, which is important to make sure you are
adequately hydrated.

The catheter bag will be emptied regularly by your nurse's aide, and
the Foley is typically removed the day after surgery. Nobody is looking at
your private parts when the bag is removed. You will be covered and given
a damp washcloth to clean away any leaks. A catheter eliminates the need
to get up and go to the bathroom, which is a difficult proposition when
you are numb and loopy.

Occasionally, a catheter may feel uncomfortable, and men in particular
are thrilled to get it out. Men can still avoid a trip to the bathroom by using
a plastic bottle called a urinal—a device so convenient that many men
take it home to use at night. Conversely, women are sometimes reluctant
to have it removed. But the risk of a urinary tract infection increases the
longer the catheter is left in. In most circumstances, the catheter is taken
out the day after surgery, by which time you will be walking not only to the
bathroom but outside in the hallway with a therapist. However, you can
also walk with a catheter, on the day of surgery, and therapists and nurses
are very accustomed to either carrying the bag or hooking it onto a walker.
The therapist who walks with you will make sure it doesn't pull or cause
discomfort when you are moving.

Compression Pumps

Surgery carries the risk of blood clots, and a prolonged period of not moving after surgery doesn't help. That is why many orthopedic surgeons want
their patients up and moving as soon as possible, within hours of awakening from anesthesia. As you lie in bed, semi-immobilized, you will feel a
rhythmic squeezing and releasing sensation from the compression devices
wrapped around your calves (or just one calf, in the case of ankle patients).
You may hear them, too; they make a humming sound.

The wraps attach via tubing to a pumping machine, a box that hooks
over the bedrail. Set to a certain pressure, the wraps inflate and deflate,
alternately squeezing and massaging your calves. Some people love the

effect of compression pumps so much that they ask to take them home. Others complain of feeling hot and annoyed by them. If your wraps feel too tight or dig into your skin, or if you think they aren't working correctly, let your nurse know. Once you are up and moving, you won't need the wraps as much. You may also be wearing white compression stockings in addition to the compression pumps, depending on your surgeon's preference.

EXTRAS FOR KNEE PATIENTS

Many surgeons use a local nerve block in addition to your spinal or general anesthesia to reduce pain around the knee. If you have such a block, you will have another tube emerging from your thigh that delivers numbing medication from a bulb-like device. The bulb will sit inside a small nylon case on your bed. If you get up and walk with a therapist while the nerve block is still active, the therapist will bring the case along. If the block has caused temporary weakness in your thigh muscles, particularly the quadriceps, a therapist may apply a knee brace to provide support when you walk. The brace is only used until you regain muscle control.

You will have ice on your knee in one form or another. One popular device is a polar care ice machine—there are various brands. The size of a small cooler—one surgeon at my hospital joked that it holds a six pack of beer cans—it delivers a continuous cold sensation into rubbery pads wrapped around your knee. The pads are attached to the cooler via tubes, and the cooler, which is plugged in to an electrical outlet, sits on the floor. The great thing about these devices is that they work for a long time, about three hours. Although not essential—and you may have to pay for it out of pocket—it is a very effective method for taking the edge off your pain. Ice, in conjunction with elevation, reduces swelling in the knee. You may be able to borrow a polar machine from a friend; just make sure the pads are clean. Always place a layer of fabric, such as a pillowcase or a cloth, between your skin and the wrap.

You may have heard of a continuous passive motion (CPM) machine.[14] This is a heavy contraption placed under your entire leg while you are in bed. It continuously bends and straightens your knee, at first just a small amount, for two hours at a time. You can turn it off with a remote, and you can also change the setting when you are ready to tolerate more bending. Some people like the feeling of having their knee moved, but CPM machines have fallen out of favor for total knee patients and are no longer universally used. Studies have shown that there is no statistical difference in knee mobility in people who do and don't use them. Plus, they are heavy and clunky, they must be fitted correctly to each patient, someone other than the patient must be taught how to use them, and renting them costs money.

Also, the more time you spend lying down with your leg in the CPM, the less time you are moving on your own. Current thinking holds that it's healthier to not only bend and straighten the knee on your own, but to get up and move. Some surgeons still use a CPM machine in certain cases, such as in a revision surgery—if part or all of an implant is removed and replaced due to a problem—or for someone with a history of excessive scar tissue formation, or for someone who tends to be sedentary. If you feel strongly that you would benefit from a CPM machine, talk to your surgeon.

EXTRAS FOR HIP PATIENTS

If you have a traditional posterior hip replacement, you may wake up with a large foam wedge lodged between your legs to keep them apart. If you recall your hip precautions, you are not allowed to cross the surgical leg over the midline of your body. The wedge insures that you can't do so. Most surgeons abandon the wedge soon after surgery, but you will need to keep your legs apart with pillows or bolsters as long as you have hip precautions.

You can still roll onto one side, as long as you have pillows to keep your legs apart. While it may seem counterintuitive, it is generally safer to roll onto the surgical side once the incisional pain subsides. If you sleep on your good side, the surgical leg on top could fall off the pillow and cross the midline of your body.

EXTRAS FOR SHOULDER PATIENTS

Regardless of whether you have a traditional or a reverse total shoulder replacement, you will likely have some form of a sling or a brace on the operated shoulder. Some surgeons require that you wear the brace at all times except during therapy; others let you remove it at will. If your nurse isn't sure about how to adjust or remove the brace, an occupational or physical therapist should be able to help.

You will also have ice on your shoulder, either in the form of ice packs or a polar care ice machine (similar to one designed for knee patients) which will have a blue wrap anatomically designed to fit the shoulder, an ice-water cooler plugged in to an electrical outlet, and tubing that attaches the two. The wrap is held in place by Velcro, which is convenient, because regular ice bags tend to fall off the shoulder. Always place a layer of fabric, such as a pillowcase or a T-shirt, between your skin and the ice wrap.

EXTRAS FOR SPINE PATIENTS

If you have a neck fusion, you may have a Miami J (or similar) hard collar to immobilize your neck, plus a separate brace, such as an Aspen collar, to wear when showering. You and your caregiver will learn how to don and doff the braces.

If you have low-back surgery, you may have a few extra attachments. These include one or two tubes delivering additional numbing medication to your surgery site—each accompanied by a black bag containing the medication in a rubber bulb—and a drain to prevent blood from pooling under the skin. You may be prescribed a back brace that provides compression and support for out-of-bed activities, but you don't have to wear this in bed. Your physical or occupational therapist will teach you how to put on the brace while sitting at the edge of the bed, without bending or twisting.

EXTRAS FOR ANKLE PATIENTS

You may not have any extra lines, but you will find your surgical foot positioned about two feet above the bed on layers of pillows. This position should feel fairly comfortable—you can also elevate your head to achieve a V-shaped position—and your ankle may feel numb. The local block you receive for surgery should last anywhere from 18 to 36 hours. Ask your surgeon how long your block will last so you can plan accordingly and take pain medication before it wears off.

ROOM EQUIPMENT

Hospital rooms usually come equipped with a few other things you would be wise to recognize.

Whiteboard

If your hospital room has a communication board, also called a white-board, and the staff is serious about using it, try to pay attention to what is written on it. A whiteboard holds information about you: your diagnosis, your precautions, and the names of your surgeon, hospitalist, nurse, and your nurse's assistant or aide, perhaps even the name and phone number of your family member, and the anticipated day of your discharge. This is important information, for you and for everyone who comes in. If someone other than your own nurse or aide takes you to the bathroom, for instance, that person needs to know your diagnosis, your weight bearing status, and any movement precautions you may have.

Some nurses also record each pain medication dose on the whiteboard, including the drug's name, the dosage, and the time it was given. Again, it is helpful for others to see this information. Let's say a therapist comes to work with you in the afternoon, and you report pain of 7/10 (that is, 7 on a scale of 1 to 10—see chapter 7). The therapist sees on the whiteboard that your last dose of pain medication was three hours ago and can ask your nurse about giving you something for *breakthrough* pain. This is a request you can also make. Breakthrough simply means you need something extra to tide you over until the next dose is due. The whiteboard lets you keep track. But this system of communication only works when everybody uses it and updates it consistently.

Gait Belt

Many orthopedic rooms also come equipped with a gait belt, a therapy tool used to keep you safe when you move. The belt will be wrapped around your waist, at your center of gravity, and held by a therapist when you stand up and walk.

Here is a short aside illustrating the merits of using a gait belt when you are walking with a therapist or other staff member. I was working with a total shoulder patient for the first time the morning after surgery. He was eager to see me, because he and his wife were raring to go home. Before he could leave, I had to make sure he knew his exercises and could move safely. The occupational therapist had already cleared him to go home, and she was marveling at how well he had done. He was dressed, with his sling on, and alert, so much so that I hesitated to put a gait belt around him. But I did; it is a matter of good procedure, like washing hands between patients. He was exceptionally tall: 6'10". The gait belt wrapped around his waist was at my chest level. I am under 5'7".

Already sitting at the edge of the bed, with all of his lines removed, he stood up very quickly and started walking fast. His wife waved at both of us with a cheery smile as he sailed away down the hall.

"Let's do the stairs," he said. He walked to the stairwell and went up and down a flight of stairs. I stayed close, but it all seemed like a formality he wanted to dispense with. At the bottom of the stairs, he paused to get a drink at the water fountain; he had to stoop over to reach it. But when he stood upright, something looked wrong. Maybe it was the way his free hand slid off the fountain. He began to crumple. I quickly grabbed him by the gait belt as he fell backward and sideways. I managed somehow to protect his head and to save his surgical shoulder from hitting the carpeted floor as he landed with a thud, his large body falling partly on top of mine. I was already yelling for help as he lost consciousness. Help arrived fast, and he was assessed by a critical care team on the floor, lifted into a wheelchair, and returned to his room.

He revived quickly and completely with IV fluids. He had to stay a few extra hours and have cardiac tests to rule out anything serious. The consensus was that he had a classic *vasovagal response*, an episode of fainting brought on by a sudden decrease in blood pressure and heart rate. This is not an uncommon occurrence after a surgery, and when it happens, there is often little or no warning; a gait belt can mean the difference between no injury and a repeat trip to the operating room. He wasn't hurt, and I wasn't either. I am sure my training with the gait belt saved him from harm. Had he been a little shorter than 6'10", I could have gently lowered him to the floor.

Most hospital falls occur when a patient gets up alone without calling or when a staff member fails to use a gait belt, especially at night when taking someone to the bathroom. Your gait belt is yours to take home. It can be a great tool for your family members to use when assisting you on stairs. After knee surgery, you can use it to help bend your knee by looping it around your foot and pulling back. After hip surgery, you can loop it around your foot and pull your surgical leg out to the side for a good stretch.

Call Buttons

The bathroom in your orthopedic hospital room should have bars in the shower and next to the toilet, as well as a call button and pull cord.

Always make sure when someone leaves your room that you have your personal call button within reach, whether you are in bed or in a chair. This should not be your responsibility, of course, but try to stay aware of its location when you are awake. The call button lets you summon help; in my hospital it was combined with the television remote.

The Lovely Hospital Gown

By now you may be wondering how you could possibly move with all of these accessories. Most of them can be detached by a nurse or a therapist. Those that can't will tag along with you. And when you first get up, you may only be wearing hospital clothing—that is, a flimsy gown. About 95 percent of orthopedic patients ask if their butt is covered when they get up; the other 5 percent say they don't care because "everyone here has seen it all before."

I once had an elderly female knee patient sitting on the edge of the bed when her surgeon knocked and came in. She quickly reached back to close the gap in her gown—I hadn't had time to tie it or give her a second gown to wrap around her back, like a cape. He didn't seem to notice—surgeons see skin and body parts all day long, after all—and he launched into an explanation of how her surgery had progressed and asked if she had questions. They talked for a couple of minutes.

As he turned to leave, he said with a smile, "Oh, and Mimi, I've seen your butt before."

"Oh," she said with a chuckle. "I guess you have."

All staff members should make sure you are entirely covered when you venture into the hallway to meet and greet your fellow gown-clad orthopedic warriors. You may bring your own gown and robe, or shorts and a T-shirt to the hospital, to exchange for the hospital gown while you still have all these lines attached, but don't bring anything really nice. Hospital clothes get stained and dirty.

Chapter 5

Who's Who in the Hospital

After you emerge from the operating room's recovery suite, still lying groggily in bed, you will be transported to your hospital room. The first people you will meet are your nurse and your certified nursing assistant. They won't expect you to do anything except lie there and relax. They will check your heart rate, blood pressure, and oxygen saturation, and monitor your pain, your sensation, urine output, bowel sounds, and your level of alertness—some of them every thirty minutes. The first few hours in your hospital room may not be as restful as you might like.

A person in a lab coat, the hospitalist, may come in soon after you arrive. The hospitalist is the doctor in charge of your medical needs. She will talk to you about any potential effects of surgery on your current health, such as a change in blood values or kidney and bladder function. If you have a chronic condition for which you take medications, such as diabetes, the hospitalist will manage it during your stay. The hospitalist is your expert resource for all medical questions.

The surgeon, the only clinician you may truly wish to see, may or may not make an appearance. If he doesn't, it's usually because he is busy in the operating room on another case. You will have many visitors and you may not remember everything that happens during this period, so this is a good time to have your spouse or companion in the room to act as another set of eyes and ears. This person should feel free to ask questions and take notes on your behalf.

After a couple of hours in your room, just as you begin to think the interruptions are surely over and you can drift back into dreamland, another pair of people may file in. They introduce themselves as a physical therapist and a rehab tech. The therapist will ask personal questions about who lives with you, how your home is configured, and how well you functioned before surgery. The rehab tech will start to disconnect your attachments. These people actually want to get you out of bed. If nobody told you they were coming, you may feel incredulous.

"Are you kidding me?" you may say. "You want me to get up now? My surgeon never told me about *this*."

I have been on the receiving end of these words so many times that I have to laugh. The surgeon is in fact the person who asked us to come in and get you walking as soon as possible. At my hospital, about half of the surgeons routinely requested physical therapy for their hip and knee patients on the day of surgery. Your nurse has told us you are alert enough, you have sensation in both legs, your vitals are stable, you aren't complaining of nausea, and your pain is under control. If you are a patient whose surgeon believes in the merits of early mobility, I consider you fortunate.

You get to walk.

Therapists are pretty thick-skinned, but because we are the ones who actually ask you to do something other than just lie there, we often become the target of unfriendly fire. Try to think of this interruption as a positive thing. You haven't moved on your own all day and your joints have stiffened. Moving may feel good. Walking reduces your risk of getting a blood clot. And you actually *can* walk on that new hip or knee, just hours after surgery. That is incredibly exciting.

Walking soon after surgery will give you a hefty dose of bravado and put you at greater ease the next time you get up. You are getting a head start on the patients who have to wait another twelve or fifteen hours to walk. And this could mean you will get to go home earlier.[15] If you are still doubtful, consider this: People who take their first walk a few hours after surgery often ask afterward, "How many more times can I do that again tonight?" They forget momentarily how exhausted they are, because they are so thrilled.

If you arrive to your room late in the day, after the therapy team has left, and you would like to get up, ask your nurse if you can get up to a chair. A dedicated nurse (and aide) will help you if there is time.

All of the health-care providers at the hospital—the nurse, the certified nursing assistant, the hospitalist, the therapy team, and others—are important players on your care team. You will see a few of them within a couple hours of your arrival. The onslaught will continue the next day. Nobody expects you to be at your best. If you can appreciate that each person is enhancing your care, doing something you actually need but may not understand, you are less likely to feel annoyed. If you understand a little about who does what, you will know better about how to direct your questions and get them answered by the right person.

Here is a more detailed description of the key providers you will see. Each one will have a name tag and should introduce himself or herself by name and specialty.

SURGEON

He (the majority of orthopedic surgeons are male) is the highly trained medical doctor who replaces your degenerated body part or fuses vertebrae in your spine. In the case of the knee surgeon, he makes the incision, removes diseased bone and cartilage, as well as ligaments you no longer need, shapes and levels the joint surfaces to accommodate the new implant pieces, and then puts the pieces in place. When finished, he sews multiple layers of tissue back together, often in concert with an assistant. The top layer of skin may be covered with a shiny glue called Dermabond, or stitched or stapled together. The surgeon works as quickly as possible to minimize blood loss and the amount of time you are under anesthesia. Shorter periods of time under general anesthesia are associated with a lower risk of complications, such as blood clots and lingering cognitive effects.

You have spoken with your surgeon before your procedure, and you are eager to see him again now that it's over. Your spouse or companion who brought you to the hospital and remained in the waiting room has already heard how the surgery went, but you may not remember. A good question to ask your surgeon, when you see him, is "did the surgery go as you expected?" The answer will tell you whether your operation was straightforward or if he encountered something unexpected.

If the surgeon says that something did not go as he expected, or he had to do more work than anticipated, ask him to explain what that means. Again, this is a good time to have your surrogate present. Otherwise, you may wait ten days or longer to talk to the surgeon again.

ANESTHESIOLOGIST

This is another highly trained physician who is responsible for your well-being during surgery. You don't get to choose your anesthesiologist, but if you are concerned, ask your surgeon about the credentials of the anesthesiologists at your hospital. The anesthesiologist assigned to you will likely call you at home the night before surgery and speak with you again in the morning in the preoperative area of the hospital. You will be asked about your medical conditions (the anesthesiologist will already have access to your records), medications, drug allergies, surgeries, and any previous adverse reaction you have had to anesthesia.

The best advice I can give is to pay close attention to the questions, answer them thoroughly, and be sure to tell your anesthesiologist of any issues you have had in the past with a surgical procedure. I once had a vasovagal response—an episode of lightheadedness and nausea brought on by a sudden decrease in blood pressure and heart rate that caused me to slump forward and briefly faint while sitting in the recovery chair—so I make sure to mention that incident with the anesthesiologist prior to any procedure. As a result, I am given extra IV fluids to keep my blood pressure from dropping precipitously. I've never had the problem again.

A spinal block, which causes complete numbness from the waist down, is used in hip, knee, and ankle surgeries. One common misconception is that if you have spinal anesthesia during your surgery, as opposed to general anesthesia, you will be awake. Not true. (There is no way you would want to watch your own joint replacement surgery, but you can watch someone else's on YouTube if you wish.) First you will receive medication in your IV to induce a form of amnesia. You will not remember anything, although you may say things and follow commands. You will not feel the needle going into your spinal region for the anesthesia. When you awaken after surgery, you will have little sense of how much time has passed.

The main advantage of a spinal block is you aren't intubated—you breathe on your own and do not need a breathing tube and a ventilator. You are also less likely to experience nausea and vomiting, and the risk of a blood clot is lower. Most knee and ankle surgeons also use a local nerve block or a strong injection into the joint to provide ongoing pain relief in the surgical region after you wake up. The spinal wears off so that you can move, but the local block or injection continues to produce a numbing effect around the surgery site. Local injections are administered by the surgeon after the anesthesiologist has placed the spinal block.

Shoulder surgeons often use a general anesthesia as well as another kind of local block, called an interscalene block, which numbs the area from the neck down through the hand. A general anesthesia must be used for spine fusion surgery. You will receive a breathing tube in your throat with general anesthesia, but you will not be awake when it is inserted. Also, if you previously had hardware placed in your lumbar spine you will be given a general anesthesia for your knee, hip, or ankle lumbar replacement, as the hardware could interfere with the insertion of the spinal.

During your actual procedure, either the anesthesiologist or a certified registered nurse anesthetist (CRNA) stays close to your head in the operating room and carefully monitors your vital functions, such as breathing, blood pressure, body temperature, heart rate, and heart rhythm. If something changes, the anesthesiologist can make adjustments in the medications, fluids, and oxygen you are receiving.

Someone from anesthesia will likely visit you in your room the day after surgery. It may not be the same person who attended your surgery, but he or she will be familiar with your case. You will have the chance to ask follow-up questions about the anesthesia that was used and any side effects you may be experiencing.

CERTIFIED REGISTERED NURSE ANESTHETIST

The certified registered nurse anesthetist (CRNA) is a registered nurse who additionally holds a minimum of a master's degree in an accredited nurse anesthesia education program. New programs now offer CRNAs a doctoral degree, and the field has grown greatly, in part because the services of CRNAs cost less than those of anesthesiologists, even though their decision-making privileges and their methods of delivering medication are the same. In 2001, the federal government, specifically the Centers for Medicare and Medicaid Services, gave states the right to decide whether CRNAs could practice without physician supervision; to date, about a third of the states have voted to allow it. In my orthopedic hospital, CRNAs work side-by-side with anesthesiologists, and either will see patients the next day. If you have any questions about the anesthesia professionals in your facility, ask your surgeon.

HOSPITALIST

Up until the 1990s, your personal physician might have come to see you in the hospital. This trend has largely disappeared, and now we have hospital doctors, called hospitalists. The field of hospital medicine is the fastest-growing specialty in the history of the profession.[16] Your personal doctor, if you have one, may be miles away from the hospital, seeing patients in an office at the very time you need care. A hospitalist is in the building with you, or close by, at all times. The hospitalist has similar training to that of an internal medicine doctor, but has more in-depth experience in specific hospital scenarios and emergencies.

If you have a history of hypertension, for instance, this physician monitors changes in your blood pressure, and adjusts your medications accordingly. The same is true of any heart and respiratory conditions, diabetes or other endocrine issues, and psychological or neurological problems. Even if you have no significant medical history and are perfectly healthy before surgery, you will still be seen by a hospitalist, sometimes before surgery if there is a question about your preoperative medical workup, such as a heart arrhythmia, and definitely afterward, at least once a day. The hospitalist is in charge of keeping you safe and stable in the immediate hours and days after surgery. He or she has studied your medical profile, knows and understands the medications you are taking, and is alert to any complications that could arise as a result of surgery.

It is very important for you and your family member to communicate openly and clearly with the hospitalist, even though you have never met this person before. You may see more than one hospitalist during your stay, although every attempt is made to keep patients with the same doctor from day to day.

In the small orthopedic hospital where I worked, one or two hospitalists were present during the day, readily accessible not only to patients but also to other clinicians. Each morning, our staff would hold a meeting, called a *huddle*, of representatives from each discipline—orthopedics, medicine (the hospitalist), pharmacy, therapy, nursing, and case management—to discuss the status of each patient. This was a good way of keeping everyone informed and updated about important developments in a patient's recovery status. You can assume when somebody new comes to see you from any discipline, such as a new nurse or therapist, that this person knows your current medical status. If you aren't sure, just ask.

ORTHOPEDIC PHYSICIAN ASSISTANT

If you have a family doctor or internist, chances are you have encountered a physician assistant (PA) in the office. A PA is often indistinguishable from a doctor and sees patients independently in a private-practice setting. A PA's training consists of two to three years of post-collegiate medical education and clinical-rotation training, similar to but less than a physician's, resulting in a master's degree in health science, medical science, or physician assistant studies. PAs must pass a state certification exam, and some pursue additional specialty training.

The PA can examine, diagnose, order tests, prescribe medications, and treat patients, as long as he or she is working as part of a team that includes physicians. The same is true in the hospital, where PAs wear lab coats and work on teams with doctors. Some orthopedic PAs assist surgeons in the operating room. Others work on the hospital floor during daytime hours as representatives of the surgeons.

Think of your PA as the surgeon's surrogate, someone to whom the surgeon has entrusted your care. The surgeon can't be in two places at once, and although he will likely make an appearance, the PA is more readily available. The PA consults with the surgeon, manages your orthopedic pain by prescribing a cocktail of medications that is unique and specific to your needs, and is primarily responsible for all your orthopedic issues. The PA also works closely with your hospitalist and your nurse. If a medication isn't working or its side effects are causing you problems, such as nausea or vomiting, the PA can act quickly to change your prescriptions.

Additionally, the PA monitors your swelling, checks for signs of complications such as a *blood clot*, and changes your wound dressing (with or without your nurse's help.)

The orthopedic PAs I have worked with are highly competent, trustworthy, and hardworking. If something isn't working for you from an orthopedic perspective, it is your prerogative to speak to the PA. This is what your surgeon expects you to do.

REGISTERED NURSE

A registered nurse (RN) will be assigned to you before you arrive on the floor after surgery. She or he will know how you progressed in the recovery room, what medications you take, and any drug allergies you have. The RN will spend a chunk of time with you when you first arrive on the floor, making sure all your lines are intact, your monitors are working, and that you are medically stable and positioned comfortably. If your room has a whiteboard, ask the nurse to write her name and hospital phone number on it if she doesn't do so voluntarily. Your name, room number, and phone number also should be written on the board. A conscientious nurse will also write your diagnosis, your precautions, and the name of your hospitalist and surgeon on the board. As noted in chapter 4, this is helpful so that you, your family or friends, and other providers can see at a glance any vital information they may need.

A person can become a registered nurse by various means, either by earning a bachelor's degree, an associate's degree, or a diploma from a nursing school.

The nurse is the point person for all other providers, the one who communicates breaking news about you to the hospitalist, the PA, and the therapy team. She or he records and interprets your blood work and vital signs, brings your medications, educates you about their purpose, watches you take them, and monitors for side effects. Depending on your hospital's policy, he may also write on the whiteboard the name of each of your medications, the time it is given, and when your next dose is due. This is particularly helpful to you with regard to pain medication, especially if you experience a sudden onset of breakthrough pain. You may not remember exactly when you received your last dose of pain medication. If it was given orally just twenty minutes earlier, the drug may need more time to take effect. If it was given three hours earlier, and your next scheduled dose is an hour away, your nurse may be able to give you something to address the breakthrough pain before your next full dose is due.

Even if nothing is written on the board about the time your pain medication was given, it is always your right to speak up if your pain is not being controlled adequately. Don't wait, don't feel guilty, don't be bashful or try to suck it up. Uncontrolled pain is like an escaped prisoner. The farther away it gets, the harder it is to capture and bring back under control.

In my experience, patient complaints about failure to adequately address their pain most often occurred during the night. I think that night nurses do not always awaken their patients to bring pain medication at regular intervals because they don't want to disturb a patient who appears to be sleeping peacefully. I highly recommend discussing this topic with your night nurse at the shift change. Hospital nurses typically work twelve-hour shifts; in my setting, their shifts were from 7:00 a.m. to 7:00 p.m. and 7:00 p.m. to 7:00 a.m. If you arrive on the floor at 3:00 p.m., you will see your day nurse the first four hours and then the night nurse will take over. Tell your nurses of any concerns you have, including your preference to be awakened for nighttime pain meds.

Both the nurse and the certified nursing assistant will come to see you regularly during your first few hours in the room. They will take care of your basic needs, such as emptying your catheter or refilling the ice in your cooler or cold pack. You will be able to order your own food, but they should make sure that your menu, your call button, your television remote, and any other devices you need are within reach and that you know how to use them.

In the unlikely event you need to use the bathroom before a therapist comes (most patients have a Foley catheter to collect urine for the first night), the nurse or certified nursing assistant can help you transfer to a bedside commode or walk to the bathroom. You and your family members should feel confident that they are familiar with your movement restrictions and precautions. If they seem unsure, remind them before they move you. They should also use a gait belt each time they help you out of bed. In an orthopedic hospital, every patient is designated a fall risk. Your wristband or sock color will attest to this—each color means something different. Some patients are at greater risk of falling than others, but falls are unpredictable.

Each nurse may be taking care of four to five patients in various stages of recovery. Just like other providers, nurses appreciate it when you can consolidate your requests and questions as much as possible so they aren't constantly on the run.

CERTIFIED NURSING ASSISTANT

The person who assists your nurse and works the same twelve-hour shift is called a Certified Nursing Assistant (CNA), or a Patient Care Assistant (PCA), or simply a nurse's aide. In the orthopedic setting, a nurse will have a CNA to help with each patient, and depending on your nurse's workload at any given moment, the CNA may spend more time with you. CNAs are often more experienced and more skilled than nurses at helping people move. While they lack the depth of knowledge about anatomy and physiology that therapists possess, they understand basic movement principles and safety precautions.

The CNA may not give medication or admit or discharge patients, but he takes vitals, tests blood sugar, removes catheters, and assists with personal care such as dressing, toileting, and bathing. Like all clinicians, he must be able to perform cardiopulmonary resuscitation (CPR) and basic first aid.

Some people earn their CNA certification first, work for a time as a CNA, and then pursue a nursing degree. To become a CNA, a person must have a high school degree or equivalent. The candidate then takes several months of coursework on patient care and must pass a certification exam.

PHYSICAL THERAPIST

A hospital physical therapist (PT) teaches you how to move correctly and safely, following the precautions for your diagnosis, and how to walk with an appropriate assistive device, such as a cane, a pair of crutches, or a walker. The therapist will review your prior medical history in the computer before seeing you, get additional information from the morning huddle, and check your current condition, level of alertness, and your pain level with your nurse before seeing you.

A typical PT visit lasts twenty to thirty minutes, with the exception of the first session, called the *evaluation*, which may last longer because of the interview portion. Before asking you to move, the PT will ask a series of questions to determine how well you functioned before surgery, what equipment you already have, and who will be helping you at home. If you had a knee, hip, or back surgery, the PT may be accompanied by an occupational therapist (OT), a rehab tech (both described below), or a CNA, to help with your lines and to keep you safe.

For most orthopedic surgeries, the physical therapist will work with you twice a day, once in the morning and once in the afternoon. PTs typically work an eight-hour or ten-hour shift during the day.

PTs teach the basic exercises for moving your knee, hip, and shoulder (see chapter 2) and write specific, time-sensitive goals for each patient. For example, if you are a knee patient with a two-day hospital stay, and you are planning to go home with your spouse, you would have a "bed mobility" goal (getting in and out of bed), a "transfer" goal (changing positions from sitting to standing and vice versa), a walking goal, and a stair goal. The goals specify the amount of assistance you will need with each task, and which device is the most suitable.

PTs will frequently ask if the person slated to help you at home can come in for family training, which includes teaching that person how to guard you on the stairs. Standing behind you as you ascend and facing you as you descend, the support person uses a railing, as you do, and holds you by the gait belt. Climbing stairs is one of the last tasks you will attempt before discharge.

A few words of advice with regard to physical therapy: if a PT assists you out of bed to a chair in the morning and tells you to call your CNA in one to two hours to help you return to bed, follow the instructions. Do not sit up in the chair for three or more hours and wait for the therapist to come back in the afternoon. If you do, you will be too tired for a meaningful PT session in the afternoon. And if you have had knee surgery, it is better for you to elevate your leg above your heart, in the bed, to reduce pain and swelling.

Likewise, if you are able to walk safely to the bathroom on your first visit with the therapist, ask the CNA or the nurse to take you the next time, rather than waste the next therapy visit repeating something you have already accomplished. You will benefit more from a novel activity such as venturing out into the hallway when the PT returns. Each PT may be assigned four or five patients, allowing for time to see each patient twice daily.

Unlike nurses and CNAs who are assigned to care for you over a twelve-hour shift, PTs account for their treatment time in fifteen-minute increments, and they must specify what you did and what you accomplished. This is not for payment purposes in most hospital scenarios—insurance usually pays a flat fee for an inpatient stay regardless of how much therapy you receive—it is to document your progress in the medical record.

Therapists come to see you with an agenda in mind, but they should also be flexible if you aren't feeling well. In an ideal scenario, the therapist will teach you a specific task or two during each session, watch you perform the task (such as standing up from a chair to your walker without losing your balance), and then check it off as a goal you have met. It sometimes takes more than one session to master a task.

When you meet all your goals, the therapist will *clear* you to go home.

All new physical therapy graduates now have doctoral degrees, usually a doctor of physical therapy (DPT) for the clinical setting (or a PhD for the academic setting), but you may see a PT with a master's or a bachelor's degree. This does not mean the person with a bachelor's degree is less qualified. Rather, it reflects the rapid evolution of academic programs within a short period of time; the person with the bachelor's degree has been practicing longer. In the 1990s, most institutions offering PT programs changed their degree requirement from a bachelor's to a master's. Then, in the early 2000s, all of them changed again, to require a doctorate degree. The curriculum is not substantially different or longer than the master's level curriculum except that it includes a mandatory research component. All PTs must pass a national licensure exam. Many also seek advanced certification in a specialty.

OCCUPATIONAL THERAPIST

Many patients ask, "What's the difference between physical therapy and occupational therapy?" And the word "occupational" leads quite a few patients to say, "You're not going to make me work, are you? I'm retired." Occupation in this context means the functional tasks and activities one performs throughout life, plus more complex ones that add meaning and purpose to life, such as writing or painting or otherwise working with the hands.

An occupational therapist (OT) teaches you how to perform what are called *Activities of Daily Living* (ADLs). These consist of the personal habits a healthy individual takes for granted, such as dressing, toileting, bathing, and grooming. Like the PT, the OT makes sure you follow your precautions.

For all of these surgeries, the OT focuses on problem solving with you and identifying and introducing devices that allow you to perform a task independently.

If you had a total hip replacement with posterior precautions, for instance, you will not be able to bend forward to put on socks or to pull up pants. The OT may show you how to use a sock aid. Likewise, if you have difficulty getting on and off a toilet seat comfortably, the therapist may recommend equipment such as a toilet seat riser or a raised seat with handlebars.

If you had a neck or a back surgery, the OT will teach you how to perform a log roll, how and when to apply any brace your doctor has prescribed, how to get dressed, and how to bathe safely.

Shoulder patients will learn how to manage their sling, get dressed, and to substitute the nonsurgical arm for tasks that require prohibited movements, such as shampooing or brushing your hair. If you need help performing an ADL, the OT will teach your caregiver how to do it while maintaining your precautions.

OTs work during the day and sometimes alongside PTs, especially during their first visit, also called the evaluation. They will ask questions about your prior status before surgery that are different from the PT's, such as "do you have a tub shower or a walk-in shower?" or "how far away from your bed is your bathroom?" or "did you need help with dressing or bathing before surgery?" If a patient has a cognitive issue or a physical disability, the OT will teach the caregiver how to supervise the ADLs.

Your OT will usually see you once a day. In some hospitals, OTs work with patients with upper-body surgeries, such as those with a cervical spine fusion or a total shoulder replacement, while PTs may not see these patients unless they have difficulty walking. They also document and account for each visit in fifteen-minute increments.

While veteran OTs have a bachelor's degree, all new OT graduates have a master's degree, some pursue a doctorate, and all must pass a national certification exam.

PHYSICAL THERAPY ASSISTANT AND OCCUPATIONAL THERAPY ASSISTANT

After a PT completes your evaluation, you may be seen subsequently by a physical therapy assistant (PTA). The same applies to the OT and the certified occupational therapy assistant (COTA). A PTA and a COTA are legally not allowed to perform the initial evaluation, set goals for a patient, or discharge a patient.

But they can execute the treatment plan set up by the PT and the OT respectively. In the orthopedic setting, the PTA may lead group activities. If the PTA is the last person to see you for discharge and determines that you have met your physical therapy goals, the PT must read and cosign the PTA's final note. The same is true of the OT and the COTA.

Each PTA and COTA is required to earn a two-year associate's degree and pass a licensure exam.

REHAB TECH

This person provides another set of hands to help the therapists and the therapy assistants. Rehab techs are often young people who aspire to attend a PT or PTA or an OT or COTA program. They have training in patient care, adaptive equipment, and safe ways of moving people. Rehab techs are also usually the individuals who deliver and custom-fit any equipment you may purchase during your stay, such as a walker, crutches, tub bench, sock aid, or other adaptive pieces.

RESPIRATORY THERAPIST

There is a respiratory therapist (RT) at the hospital twenty-four hours a day, an indication of this person's vital role. In the event of a critical incident, such as cardiac arrest, the RT is a first responder.

In normal circumstances, the RT monitors and interprets oxygen levels in your blood at various times during the day and during different activity demands, such as sleeping versus walking.

As noted earlier, you will wake up from surgery with a piece of clear, soft, forked tubing in your nostrils. The tubing, called a nasal cannula, delivers a specific quantity of oxygen, measured in liters per minute. Your body may need extra oxygen for a day or two after surgery, especially if you have a preexisting condition such as sleep apnea or a breathing disorder, but sometimes even if you don't.

The RT may walk alongside you during a therapy session to monitor your oxygen levels while you exercise or climb stairs. If your oxygen saturation drops below 88 percent while you are at rest, or to the low 80s with exertion, the RT may increase your oxygen level. Breathing in extra oxygen through the nasal cannula should bring the saturation up to the low or mid-90s.

It is not uncommon for healthy people to go home with an order for supplemental oxygen, especially at altitude. You needn't be alarmed if this happens; if you didn't use oxygen before surgery at home, it is unlikely you will need it for very long afterward.

CASE MANAGER

This person, often a social worker with a master's degree in social work (MSW), oversees your hospital stay and your discharge plan. If you have a strong social network, such as a family or a set of friends who can help, you may only see the case manager once. She will check to make sure you have someone to take you home from the hospital and stay with you.

If you have a doctor's order for home physical therapy after a knee replacement, the case manager will make the arrangements. She will ask if you have a preferred home health company; if you don't, she will provide names of agencies that serve your geographic area. Once you choose one, she will contact the agency and provide pertinent information about you, including your name, address, phone number, age, diagnosis, a summary of your hospital stay, an order from the surgeon, and your insurance information.

If you don't know of a good home health agency in your area, you might want to research this ahead of surgery by asking friends or your primary care physician for a recommendation.

Conversely, if you live alone, or if there is a possibility you will need to go to a sub-acute rehabilitation facility—typically the same as a skilled nursing facility (SNF)—the case manager will give you a list of places that are contracted with your insurance and ask you to choose one. She will then contact the facility on your behalf to check for an available room. One thing a case manager cannot do is reserve a bed for you ahead of surgery.

In Denver, a couple of sub-acute facilities had an excellent reputation, and patients who anticipated they would need a SNF could tour them before admission. This was facilitated by my hospital's case managers, who proactively called patients to discuss their discharge plan. If you don't have access to a case manager or a care coordinator at your hospital and you think a SNF is in your post-op future, you can contact your insurance company and ask for a list of facilities in your network.

If you have a managed care insurance policy, the nicest facilities may not be included in your network. People who came to our hospital as repeat customers and who had stayed at an inferior facility after a previous surgery often vowed never to return to "that place," because they found it depressing, lacking in therapy services, or otherwise unsatisfactory. Again, the case manager can steer you to the available rehabilitation facilities in your insurance network and help you do your homework up front. She will set up transportation from the hospital and inform you of out-of-pocket costs. But it is up to you to get informed about your options before surgery.

CHAPLAIN

Most hospitals offer the services of a spiritual or religious counselor such as a chaplain. If you are having a difficult time and would like to talk to a good listener, feel free to ask your nurse if someone is available. You don't have to be a member of any particular religious faith to ask a spiritual counselor to come and talk with you.

NURSE MANAGER

You may or may not see the nurse manager. In our hospital, a nurse manager tried to visit each patient at least once during the stay to ask if everything was okay. Sometimes nurse managers have other titles, such as lead nurse, clinical coordinator, or charge nurse, and there may be a hierarchy of several such nurses, depending on the size of your facility.

The nurse manager oversees the day-to-day operations on the floor. She is responsible for scheduling and providing adequate nursing staff, and for helping the floor nurses, hospitalists, and other staff members with questions and issues. If you have a concern about a nurse or another staff member or about your treatment plan, ask to speak to the nurse manager. If you are told there isn't one, ask to see the person in charge on the floor.

OTHER VISITORS

If you have surgery in a small specialty hospital like mine, you may also receive a visit from the chief executive officer (CEO), usually a day or two after surgery. You will also see food-service people multiple times daily and someone from housekeeping two to three times a daily. My hospital offered a massage therapist.

The most unpleasant interruption for most people comes from the phlebotomist, a person who draws your blood, usually very early in the morning. The reason for this timing is that the hospitalist needs the results of your blood work at the start of the new day. Blood is monitored carefully after surgery to check for critical changes, such as low hematocrit, which could signal the need for a transfusion.

If you crave privacy or you are an introvert and think you will become overwhelmed by all the interruptions, you may want to consider a few things. First, limit your own personal visitors from family members and friends to just one or two a day, except for a spouse or partner. If you decide you have had enough company after thirty minutes, tell them politely that you would like to sleep and ask them to leave. Also, if a clinician comes in to see you during a friend's visit, ask the friend to take a seat in the background or else step out until the clinician is finished.

If you are simply exhausted or overwhelmed, ask the nurse to put up a Do Not Disturb sign on your door for a couple of hours. This alerts other providers and personal visitors to check with your nurse before coming in. However, if a test such as an x-ray or ultrasound has been ordered, the technician may need to interrupt. This is because each hospital has a limited number of such machines, and they are in high demand.

No matter who comes in and how often, each person should always knock first. Nobody wants to disrupt your rest time, but sometimes it is unavoidable. The interruptions will bother you less if you appreciate that each person has an important job to do.

Chapter 6

Personal Demons

The following is a cautionary tale about a patient and her spouse whose actions resulted in an unnecessarily difficult first experience with physical and occupational therapy.

My occupational therapist colleague Jenny and I were assigned to see a new lumbar spine fusion patient. Kim, a woman in her forties, had undergone surgery the day before, and we had standard orders from the surgeon to work with her, meaning we were supposed to get her out of bed and walking. At 10:00 a.m., we conferred with her nurse, who gave us the green light. Kim had taken her medications at 9:00 a.m.

The moment Jenny and I entered the room, Kim burst into tears.

"I wanted to wait until noon to get my lorazepam," she sobbed. "But I know I have to do this, too."

"How are you girls today?" she then asked giddily.

She was fidgety, and what we call emotionally labile, tearing up one moment and laughing the next. I sensed a red flag, but I couldn't pinpoint what it was.

Lorazepam is the generic name for Ativan, a powerful drug used to treat anxiety. We knew that Kim, like many people, had a history of panic attacks. She had received her lorazepam at 9:00 a.m, so our timing for working with her should have been perfect. Plus, she was rating her back pain at a low level, a 3 out of 10 (see chapter 7).

Kim had not attended our preoperative spine class, where she would have learned that therapists would be coming this morning. She had never heard of a log roll (which she also would have learned in class.) We chalked up some of her anxiety to her lack of preparedness.

"You might feel better if you get up and move a little," Jenny said with a smile.

We were gentle and reassuring with her, but firm about our mission. We spent several minutes explaining what we were doing and why, asking questions about her support at home (her husband was in the building, but had temporarily left the room). She was lying on her back, and we slowly detached her lines. She finally agreed to try.

"Now, go ahead and bend your knees up," Jenny said, describing the beginning of the log roll. "Cross your arms and then roll toward me." Jenny was standing on Kim's right side, the direction she was rolling toward, and I stood on the left, ready to use the bed sheet to gently roll her body toward Jenny. (We often have to help patients the first couple of times, especially if they have been laying in one position all night and are very stiff.)

I rolled her very slowly toward Jenny, but she resisted the movement, and let out a single piercing yell, not of pain, but of fear. We paused for a few moments to let her realize she was okay. She was lying safely on her right side, facing Jenny. To help bring her upright, Jenny slowly reached forward to support Kim by the shoulders and assist her from side lying to sitting. All of a sudden, Kim sank her teeth into Jenny's right bicep.

"Did I bite you? Oh, I did, didn't I?" Red teeth marks stood out on Jenny's fair-skinned arm.

Jenny looked at her arm and said the skin wasn't broken. She chose to proceed.

Just then, Kim's husband walked in, and said, "What are you doing to her? Isn't it a bit extreme to be doing this so soon?"

"You don't have to do this now, honey," he said to Kim. "This can wait. It's not that important. Whatever it is they're doing can wait."

While it is nice to think that your spouse has your back in the hospital, it's also important to understand that prescribed orders are in place to promote a successful recovery. In this case, Kim's husband had not attended the spine class, either, and was as uninformed about the hospital routine as she was. Jenny held firm and said she would like to finish the session by getting Kim out of bed and at least up to a chair. The husband stormed out of the room.

We taught Kim how to stand up to a walker and take a few steps in it before sitting down into a straight-backed chair. We left her with her call light in hand. We instructed her to call in one hour for the nurse and CNA to assist her back to bed. At the end of the session, Kim said she felt good about getting up to the chair. She had accomplished what she needed to do, but the process didn't have to be so stressful.

Jenny and I talked to Kim's nurse, who was also caught off guard by the extent of Kim's apparent dependency on lorazepam. She was giving Kim a small dose of lorazepam every three to four hours. But Kim was apparently habituated and needed a higher dose than that after surgery. Whether it would have been safe to give her more at this time was not my call, but had the surgeon, the hospitalist, and the nurse known about the extent of her prior lorazepam habit, something could have been done. We could have waited until the afternoon, with the surgeon's blessing. Kim may have been calmer, and Jenny would not have been bitten.

When patients don't speak truthfully or fail to divulge important things, everybody suffers. While hands-on providers such as nurses and therapists typically bear the brunt of this kind of incident, the ultimate victims are the patients themselves. Once Kim's needs became more transparent, she was able to make faster progress with considerably less stress.

All of us have our personal idiosyncrasies. Most of these can be addressed easily in the hospital. If you prefer your door be left open because you are claustrophobic, that is easy to accommodate. If you prefer dim versus bright light, just say the word. I had one patient who asked us emphatically not to knock on his door, but just to come in. He had his nurse put up a sign on the door, and he got irritated and chastised the person who inadvertently knocked, out of habit.

"Please, I would prefer it if you just come in," he said with an exasperated sigh. We didn't need to understand why, but when everyone did as he asked, everything worked out. It is helpful when people share their preferences, as quirky as they may seem.

In addition to our harmless quirks, however, we have unhealthy habits, some of which we may not be proud of, but we are not ready or able to give them up. Examples of these habits include smoking, drinking (too much), eating (too much or too little), and taking illicit drugs, prescription or otherwise. Some of these habits have deep roots, origins in neglect, abuse, or other trauma, experiences that cause severe emotional pain, and affect our sense of self-worth. Life hits (almost) everyone hard at one point or another; we all bear our scars, to varying degrees.

Underlying some of these lifestyle habits can be actual psychological diagnoses, many of which are shunned by our culture as mere weaknesses and not adequately addressed: depression, bipolar disorder, anxiety disorder, obsessive compulsive disorder, post-traumatic stress disorder, eating disorder, etcetera. Our lifestyle habits can make us feel ashamed, and we often try to hide them or downplay their significance in front of others. This is not a good strategy in the hospital.

My point is this: if you can share even a little bit about these things to your personal hospital providers, you will be aptly rewarded in better treatment and more compassionate care. The staff will appreciate your honesty. It is much easier to treat what we know rather than spend time speculating about how to address odd behaviors, such as Kim's.

And the hospital in this scenario is exactly the wrong place to confront these problems and behaviors, or to pretend they don't exist. You do not want to go through a major orthopedic surgery *and* go through drug or alcohol withdrawal at the same time. Not only can this be very taxing on you and your caregivers, it can be dangerous. Going through sudden alcohol withdrawal can cause a severe and even fatal reaction.

So what's the right course of action? Just come clean about it. There is no need to be ashamed or remorseful. Look your surgeon and your hospitalist and your nurse in the eye and say, "I take narcotics regularly," or "I drink a fifth of vodka or two six packs a day," or "I am bipolar and am not on medications," or "I have PTSD." Whatever may be troubling you, even if there's not a name to it, every experienced medical team has seen it or something like it. The most likely response on the part of the physician is to address it and move on, without passing judgment. The medical team will do everything in its power, such as giving a prescribed amount of alcohol to an alcoholic in the hospital, to avoid the risk of withdrawal while a person is also coping with the normal aftermath of surgery. You might be surprised by how much kindness comes your way because of your honesty.

Rather than make anyone feel guilty, I would like to offer simple, straightforward information about some of the common habits that can and do affect recovery from a major orthopedic surgery.

EXCESSIVE DRINKING

If you drink alcohol, report the amount accurately when asked. People often underreport the amount they drink, so much so that medical providers in my orthopedic hospital routinely doubled the number that patients reported if they suspected a problem. If you say you drink rarely, but in fact you drink to excess regularly, you could be in trouble in two different ways.

First, studies show that heavy alcohol use can damage every major organ in your body, including the brain, heart, stomach, liver, pancreas, and kidneys.

A study conducted by physicians at Stanford University showed that men at the Palo Alto Veterans Affairs Hospital undergoing a hip or knee replacement who drank excessive alcohol had a greater incidence of complications after surgery, including pneumonia, stroke, gastrointestinal bleeding, blood clots, abnormal heart rhythms, urinary tract infections, surgical site infection, and delirium.[17] These are serious and costly problems that can prolong a hospital stay, lead to readmission and significantly delay recovery.

What constitutes excessive alcohol use?[18] There are a few different definitions, depending on the source. The National Institute on Alcohol Abuse and Alcoholism states that women should not consume more than one alcoholic drink daily and men not more than two. One alcoholic drink consists of one beer, one glass of wine, or 1.5 ounces of hard liquor. Other estimates are slightly more liberal, up to two drinks daily for women and three for men. Women have lower limits because they are generally smaller than men and have less water in their bodies, making them more prone to higher blood alcohol levels. But the only person who truly knows how much you drink and whether it's too much is you. One favor you can do yourself if you drink heavily is to make a serious effort to cut back during the month before surgery.

Here is the second way you can get in trouble. Let's say you drink heavily and you don't tell your medical providers. When your body expects alcohol and doesn't get it, within five to ten hours after you would normally start drinking, your heart rate, blood pressure, and breathing rate all increase. Your hands shake, you sweat more, and your body temperature increases; you feel nauseous and may vomit, and you are anxious and even agitated. Some of these symptoms, such as changes in heart rate and blood pressure, or nausea and vomiting, mimic the normal symptoms you could experience after orthopedic surgery. But the reasons for the symptoms are different, and so is the treatment.

A small percentage of people going through alcohol withdrawal will have seizures and delirium tremens (DTs), with hallucinations, severe confusion and disorientation, and heart or metabolic problems that can be life threatening. If this sounds scary, it is. But measures can be taken, including giving alcohol, when providers are able to identify the true cause of these symptoms.

To identify the complications associated with alcohol withdrawal, doctors and nurses use the Clinical Institute Withdrawal Assessment (CIWA, pronounced *see-wah*).[19] This reliable scale measures the severity of ten different symptoms associated with alcohol withdrawal. In addition to the symptoms noted above, these include tactile disturbances such as itching, hearing and visual disturbances, a specific type of headache, and cognitive disorientation. High scores on the CIWA indicate that the patient is suffering severe withdrawal symptoms and is at risk for the DTs.

Here's another reason to cut back on alcohol if you drink heavily. While orthopedic surgeons are making major efforts to reduce the use of narcotics, in favor of more localized modalities and the use of IV or injectable non-narcotic medications, most people still need at least a few doses of narcotics after surgery, especially during the first week. Alcohol, especially in large amounts, is not safe to mix with narcotics. The risks of using them together include severe breathing problems and even death.

Finally, excessive alcohol use is associated with a higher incidence of complications requiring readmission to the hospital.

SMOKING

If you smoke cigarettes, your surgeon will encourage you to quit or at least to cut back. Some spine surgeons may refuse to operate on smokers. Smoking impairs blood circulation, putting you at greater risk of wound infection. Many studies have showed that smokers who undergo a total hip replacement have a higher risk of wound infection than heavy drinkers.[20] Smoking also puts you at greater risk for breathing problems after surgery and for heart attack.[21] If you cannot quit, you can get a nicotine patch in the hospital, but you will not be allowed to smoke.

If you are interested in quitting, talk to your surgeon about the optimal time to do so. In my experience, many people reported they had quit smoking the day before surgery. A bad idea. My colleagues and I observed that this inevitably made them excessively irritable and anxious during their hospital stay. According to the website, www.strongforsurgery.com, people who quit seventy-two hours or less before surgery "may have increased secretions and more reactive airways which may interfere with anesthesia." The website suggests that smokers generally should quit at least two weeks before surgery, but should discuss their case with their surgeon.

If you live in a state where medical or recreational marijuana is legal, you may be curious about its use in the hospital. Smoking of any kind is not allowed in the hospital. But a capsule form of synthetic marijuana, Marinol, is used in medical settings to treat nausea and vomiting in cancer patients, and weight loss and anorexia in AIDS patients. I have seen Marinol used in the orthopedic setting for pain, albeit rarely. If this is an option you wish to explore, talk to your surgeon ahead of time.

OBESITY

In medical arenas, including hospitals, clinicians categorize body weight in terms of Body Mass Index (BMI).

If you would like to calculate your BMI, all you need to do is enter your height and weight into the equation provided at the Centers for Disease Control's website: www.cdc.gov/healthyweight/assessing/bmi/adult_bmi/english_bmi_calculator/bmi_calculator.html. Or you can search Google for Adult BMI Calculator.

A normal BMI falls between 18.5 and 24.9.[22] If your number falls below 18.5, see the next section on malnutrition. A number between 25 and 29.9 is considered overweight. A number of 30 or higher is considered obese. A number of 40 or higher is considered morbidly obese. A number of 50 or higher is considered super obese.

Obesity has risen dramatically in the United States, and so has the need for joint replacement. Which comes first? Does obesity cause greater arthritis? Yes. More weight means more wear and tear on the joints. Can arthritis lead to obesity in people who have difficulty exercising due to pain? Yes. People who can't walk without pain are less likely to enjoy exercising and probably less likely to do so.

Here's the rub: obesity puts a person at greater risk of complications after surgery, and the greater the obesity, the greater the risk.

One study in the *Journal of Arthroplasty* investigated the correlation between obesity and complications in the first thirty days after surgery in 13,250 total knee and total hip patients. They found that obesity was linked to a greater incidence of both superficial and deep-wound infection, the need for a return to the operating room, and a longer length of stay.[23]

Another study, performed at the Mayo Clinic in Rochester, Minnesota, and published in the *Journal of Bone & Joint Surgery*, looked at BMI in 16,136 patients who had 22,289 knee replacements over the period between 1985 and 2012.[24] The authors found a correlation between a BMI over 35 and increased infection as well as a higher need for a second surgery, called a revision, due to loosening of the prosthesis and wearing out of the plastic spacer. They also found that complications increased with higher BMI.

How you proceed if you fall into one of these categories is very much a personal and private decision that requires a heart-to-heart discussion with your surgeon. Some surgeons and groups may avoid operating if they suspect a complicated outcome. Others who have more experience operating on individuals with obesity may feel more comfortable about their track record of successful outcomes. Some surgeons may ask patients to lose weight before they will attempt surgery. Your surgeon may ask about your intentions with regard to your weight if you are morbidly or super obese. If you have no intention of trying to lose weight, and you want the surgery for pain relief, you may be disappointed in the long run when the need arises for a revision surgery. Revision surgeries for a total hip in particular can be difficult, and if your surgeon senses that you have given up on weight control, he may not want to operate.

MALNUTRITION

Being underweight, with a BMI of less than 18.5, also puts you at greater risk of complications following a total knee or total hip replacement. When comparing normal-weight and underweight individuals, a study published in the *Journal of Arthroplasty* found that among those having a hip replacement, underweight people suffered more from anemia and cardiac complications and required a longer length of stay. [25]

Among knee patients, the underweight group experienced more anemia and had a greater likelihood of developing a *hematoma*, a pooling of blood that has leaked out of the vessels and into the tissues, creating a hard, rubbery mass. The underweight group was also more likely to need a skilled nursing facility after discharge.

Regardless of the reasons for being underweight, it is a good idea to ask your surgeon if you are at greater risk for complications such as these.

OPIOID USE

"I don't want to take narcotics," you may say. "I'm afraid I'll get addicted." Many patients try to avoid taking any opiate drugs when having a joint or spine surgery because of this fear. While the likelihood of becoming addicted is small, it is real, especially for people who have a history of addiction. Fortunately, there is also a much greater awareness of the risks of addiction, and orthopedic surgeons are cutting back significantly on opioid prescriptions and turning instead to less risky alternatives, including potent combinations of IV nonsteroidal anti-inflammatory drugs and acetaminophen and the addition of other medications Most people cannot imagine taking opioid narcotics any longer than absolutely necessary because of the side effects, which can include nausea, vomiting, itching, confusion, respiratory depression, and constipation. However, if there is ever a time when you may need narcotics, it is after orthopedic surgery. It is a good idea to share your concerns and discuss your surgeon's strategy for addressing pain in a preoperative visit.

If you are already taking narcotics—such as Vicodin or Percocet or morphine—around the clock, you have likely developed at least a tolerance, if not a dependency.[26]

There are at least two problems that can arise with this scenario and orthopedic surgery. First, your body will require a higher dose of narcotics to achieve pain relief after this orthopedic surgery. This greater need increases the risk of overdose. Therefore, you need to talk to your surgeon and your hospital providers very honestly about which drugs you take and their dosage. If possible, you should decrease the use of narcotics for several weeks leading up to surgery.

Second, if you are already a chronic user, your recovery will be tougher, and you are at greater risk of staying on the drugs after this new episode of pain has resolved. One study of ongoing opioid use showed that 53 percent of total knee patients and 35 percent of total hip patients who took opioids before surgery were still using them six months later, even if their joint pain was gone.[27] Nobody should need opiates for this length of time after a successful total joint surgery. At the two-month mark, if not sooner, most orthopedic patients can cut back to one or two pills, or eliminate them completely.

Physicians recognize the opioid epidemic, and are partly responsible for causing it (see chapter 7). If you have an opiate problem and are willing to discuss it, your physician and surgeon should treat you with compassion and help you devise a strategy to address it.

A (MOSTLY) HAPPY STORY

"She hears voices, and she punched her sister last night [after surgery]," said the supervising physical therapist who attended the morning huddle. "So don't go in there alone."

"She" was Amy, a 45-year-old woman who had undergone a total knee replacement the day before. Amy had a diagnosis of schizoaffective disorder, which consists of both schizophrenia—a serious cognitive disorder—and a mood illness such as depression or bipolar disorder.

Amy was one of my new patients that day. The occupational therapist assigned to her, Mindy, was young, petite, and pregnant. She had not yet worked with a total joint patient with a significant mental illness.

"What's our strategy?" Mindy asked. She was understandably nervous. I volunteered to do the talking for both of us to avoid overstimulating the patient and to protect Mindy.

Amy was lying with the head of the hospital bed elevated. She had the blank, fixated stare of someone taking heavy doses of psychotropic drugs. While Mindy remained near the door, I approached the foot of the bed, way out of punching range, and made eye contact with Amy. I introduced both of us and spoke softly and slowly to her, asking simple questions that required only a yes or no answer. Amy's eyes locked onto mine.

"You have a really pretty smile," she said. So far, so good.

When I felt I had won enough trust to move closer, I asked Amy if it would be okay if I removed the polar ice pack from her knee. She nodded. She understood what we were doing, and she was willing to participate. I knew this could change, but she appeared calm and even engaged.

I continued to speak softly and to repeat instructions when Amy stared blankly or appeared not to follow. To my surprise, once I had removed her ice and various lines, Amy maneuvered quite easily toward the edge of the bed, without help. Her age was in her favor. All she said for three minutes was that she felt "strange." I explained that the blood was moving from her head to her feet. I asked if it was okay for us to wrap the gait belt around her waist because it would help keep her safe. Mindy moved in to one side of Amy, while I stood on the other.

"This feels weird," Amy said as she took a few steps in her walker and sat down in the waiting bedside chair. This comment was no different from what anyone else would say. The session was pleasantly uneventful. Amy remained calm throughout.

That afternoon I went back to see Amy on my own. She remembered me, but she was quieter and less responsive, as if struggling to follow my conversation. I asked about her pain, but she didn't answer. I waited.

"I'm sorry," she said. "I'm hearing voices." Since I knew it was customary for her to hear voices, I wasn't overly concerned. She was able to acknowledge it and move on.

"Can you repeat the question?" she asked.

"Sure, I asked how much pain you're having." I sat down on Amy's bed, explaining what I wanted to do. She said her pain wasn't too bad. With her permission, I gently bent her left knee, adding that it would hurt a little at first, but then it would feel looser. Then I applied a brace to her knee for added support, and directed her to the edge of the bed.

"It feels weird," she said. "I don't know how else to describe it." I placed the gait belt around her waist and showed her how to stand up without pulling on the walker. Amy was too afraid to venture out in the hallway, so I walked her around the room several laps and then assisted her into the comfortable recliner I had prepared. I elevated her legs.

I told her she had done well, and said goodbye to her for the day. She had been a superstar. And nobody (other than her unfortunate sister) got punched or bitten.

While schizoaffective disorder would be harder to conceal than a drug habit, Amy's hospital experience was much less stressful for everyone involved than Kim's. We were able to take Amy's diagnosis into account when we treated her and to make appropriate adjustments. We didn't have that chance with Kim.

One more suggestion: if you or a loved one develops a rapport with a particular provider, for any reason, don't be afraid to ask if that person can be your nurse or your therapist the next day. You may not get what you wish—that person may not be working or may be assigned elsewhere—but it can't hurt to try. I have found that for people who have special needs, or a history of abuse, or a tragic story in their lives, the continuity of care can help reduce their anxiety and allow them to focus more easily on the task at hand.

Chapter 7

Coping with Pain

The orthopedic hospital where I worked was small, and over a five-year period, I saw a lot of repeat patients. Someone would have her first knee replaced, and six weeks or six months later she would return to have the other knee done.

"This is so much easier the second time around," the majority of the "repeats" would say. "I don't have nearly as much pain." I was happy for them, yet I wondered *Why is that?* Did the surgeon do something different this time? Possibly. Did the staff have a better handle on this person's pain management the second time? Maybe. But if the patient had the same excellent surgeon, and the same excellent post-op care, was there something about the patient that made the second experience easier?

There were a few patients who had the opposite experience, reporting that surgery was harder the second time around. They said they "didn't remember" having so much pain during their first admission. They wouldn't come right out and say, "I had less pain the first time," or "I have more pain this time." They usually said they "didn't remember." This, too, intrigued me, because many people are medicated to the point that they truly do not remember much about their hospital experience.

I once saw an acquaintance at the first Denver hospital where I worked, who had both of her knees replaced there. Beth was a likable woman with a big heart, and when I learned she was there, I went to her room to say hi. She was receiving physical therapy with a colleague of mine on the acute orthopedics floor, who saw her twice daily for three days. After that, Beth continued her recovery in our rehab unit.

I ran in to Beth again some years later. She remembered seeing me in the hospital. But then she claimed that she didn't have any therapy until she went to the rehab unit.

"Sure you did," I countered. "That's where I saw you. You worked with Mary. I saw you taking steps with her in the hall. She saw you twice a day. That was the acute inpatient unit."

Beth didn't remember any of it. She insisted she didn't have any therapy until she went to the rehab unit. She didn't have dementia or any other memory impairment. But she did have significant pain in both knees and she was commensurately medicated during her inpatient stay. The entire experience was a blur to her. I have seen the same thing happen with many other patients. They either had very poor recollection of their inpatient experience, or they specifically told me that they "never had any therapy in the hospital the last time." If the hospital experience can affect patients' memory of events like therapy, might it also affect their memory of pain?

WHAT'S YOUR PAIN PROFILE?

Pain is so subjective and so individual, that almost every discussion about it is debatable or controvertible. It is easy to identify the pain medications and explain how they work differently, but it's much harder to say, "this is how this particular drug will work for you." The same is true of the side effects. Unless you can recall a specific response to a drug such as Percocet, for instance, neither you nor your physician knows how well it will work for you and whether the typical side effects (nausea, vomiting, dizziness, altered mental status, itchiness) will affect you. The one nearly universal side effect is constipation, so everybody who gets opioids for pain also gets stool softeners in the hospital.

There are two take-home messages here. First, the more you know about pain meds you have taken before and how you have responded to them, the better. Just as you may have a penicillin allergy, it is also possible to have an adverse response to narcotics, or just one narcotic. If you know you didn't

tolerate Percocet but you did well with Dilaudid or Ultram, this is important to share with your doctors and nurses. Second, let's contemplate why
someone's second knee replacement might be "easier" than the first, when
both were done by the same surgeon and in the same setting.

If you have already been through a total knee replacement and you
had a positive outcome, you are aware of what to expect. You had ups and
downs while going through therapy and the recovery process, but all in all,
it was worthwhile, and you have come back for the second knee. Coming
back for the second knee, you are probably less fearful of the pain. Because
you came through the first surgery successfully, you are more confident
that you will do so again. There is less anxiety attached to the pain. Indeed,
patients who return after their first successful joint surgery often say their
only regret is that they didn't do it sooner.

How you approach pain and how you cope with it are very important. I have a friend who recently had a complex ankle surgery to correct a
congenital defect—called an accessory navicular bone—that was causing
pain. Her surgery took several hours, longer than most total joint replacements, and the recovery was painful. When she had the twenty-five staples
removed, the ankle stretched and casted in a new position; this, too, hurt
a lot.

"My foot wasn't too happy about it," she said. "But I am happy with
the progress."

I admired the way she could isolate the foot from the rest of her body
and from her overall well-being, and also how she could take the long view
about her progress. I found her approach to pain very healthy.

An opposite approach, an unhealthy one, would be to catastrophize
your pain, a phenomenon that has been studied in orthopedic patients.
Someone who catastrophizes their pain after knee surgery may say something like, "I don't think it's supposed to hurt this much; there must be
something wrong." This person may worry that the pain means something
terrible is happening to them.

The term "pain catastrophizing" was defined in 1987 by Aaron Beck,
PhD, as "a maladaptive cognitive style originally seen in patients with anxiety and depressive disorders with an irrational negative forecast of future

event."[28] Please do not misinterpret this to think that I am suggesting that the pain is all in your head. The pain is real. But you have considerable control over what your brain does with the pain messages.

PAIN = HEALING

Pain is your body's normal response to an injury, and surgery is injurious. When you have been cut through all layers of the skin, the fascia, the muscle, and into the bone—all of which have copious nerve endings to transmit pain signals to your brain—your body responds to this injury by sending protective chemicals and blood cells to investigate. These cells, in rushing to protect the injury, actually cause more pain (in the form of heat and swelling), but they also initiate the recovery process. As contradictory as it seems, pain means your body is starting to heal.

"I tell patients that the pain they are experiencing now is the pain of recovery, and it will get better," says Dr. Foran, OrthoColorado's director of total joint replacements. "The arthritis pain that they had was the pain of the disease and was only going to get worse."

The person who has a healthy attitude toward pain recognizes that it is normal and says to herself, "this isn't fun, but I know it's supposed to happen and there's no point in fighting it. I can live with a certain level, I know it's going to get better, and the meds can help handle the worst part." This person, rather than complaining "my surgeon never told me it would hurt this much," accepts the pain and works with it. She will try to put it someplace in her psyche where it doesn't overwhelm her.

I once had a psychologist as a patient who was very good at handling her pain after a knee replacement. She was a meditator who spoke articulately about how her practice calmed her. Somehow, she smiled and seemed to be able to transcend the pain. Her serenity impressed me so much that I bought the book she recommended, *Buddha's Brain: The Practical Neuroscience of Happiness, Love & Wisdom*, by Rick Hanson, PhD. The book discusses how the neuronal connections in our brain actually change based on the repetitive patterns that our mind feeds the brain. It stands to reason that this capacity of the brain to develop new connections can work to our advantage if we harness the mind to link pain and the healing process in a positive way.

The psychologist took pain meds on schedule, and she communicated calmly with the staff. Each time I worked with her, she was gracious, friendly, and in control of her emotions.

I also saw military personnel who seemed to handle orthopedic pain very well. I think it is because of several things. They had endured physical hardship before, in basic training at the very least, and often in real and threatening situations. And they had experienced and learned to cope with severe mental stress as well. Perhaps because of this history of hardship, they were able to put their injury into perspective by saying to themselves, "this, too, shall pass."

This should not be misinterpreted as a call to act tough or underreport pain. But these patients took ownership of their pain. They didn't blame anyone for it (and they didn't take it out on hospital staff). If they felt they were close to needing a dose of medication, they would simply say so and call their nurse. I don't think achieving a state of mental toughness requires a stint in the military. People attain it in different ways.

There are affirmative breathing techniques, meditation, massage, music therapy, and other ways of coping with the emotional aspect of pain. If you think any of these alternative therapies would help, ask if your hospital offers them. And bring your own music or meditation files or CDs with you to the hospital.

THE PAIN SCALE

Now that you have learned about the emotional factors to contemplate with regard to pain, and how to enlist your own best coping strategies, here's one very easy thing to understand: the pain scale.

The pain scale is a visual analog scale, meaning it is like a ruler with the numbers 0 through 10 interspersed at equal intervals.[29] A 1 or a 2 constitute mild pain. At my hospital, the goal after surgery was to keep a patient's pain at a 3. The complete elimination of pain so early in the process is not realistic. If your doctor promises otherwise, he is doing you a disservice. A pain of 3 is low enough to allow for sleep. Trying to eliminate pain completely—except with local injections into the joint given during surgery that keep the site numb for a number of hours—would mean you would be too drugged to get up and move, which as you know by now, is important.

If you cannot use the visual analog scale due to vision impairment, or if you are caretaking a patient who may be incapable of using it, there is also a comparable "faces" scale for quantifying pain. The faces scale was developed for children and is usually displayed along with the visual analog pain scale somewhere in your hospital room.

You will be asked frequently, as many as ten times a day after surgery, "What is your pain on a scale of zero to ten?" You may become annoyed by this question, and tempted to respond, "It just hurts, okay?!" But providers want to get specific feedback so they can adjust your care accordingly. It also doesn't help if you say your pain is an 11 or a 20, especially if you are making a joke about it. A 10 is like labor pain at its worst or the pain of being severely burned; you will be in distress if your pain reaches a 10. Your blood pressure and heart rate will rise, and you will feel desperate for relief. Use the pain scale to your benefit; take it seriously.

Pain can and does creep up at times, especially at night. It is very important to notify your nurse as soon as this happens, even if you received pain medications thirty minutes earlier. There is usually something that can be done, such as repositioning, icing, walking, or supplementing a pain pill with a muscle relaxer. Remember, it is much easier to treat pain before it gets out of control.

THE OPIOID CONTROVERSY

Many people are confused by the names and the types of pain medicine. Adding to that confusion is the current controversy about opioid use. A little history is worth knowing. In the late 1990s, there was a groundswell of support for a measure that would make pain the "fifth vital sign." The other four vital signs are heart rate, blood pressure, respiratory rate, and temperature. The movement to take pain more seriously emerged from the VA hospital system in the late 1990s, and for the past fifteen years, hospitals in particular have made greater efforts to quantify pain and address it.[30]

However, that same movement to better address pain—and to improve patient satisfaction scores—led to overprescribing of opioid pain medications, which are highly addictive. Deaths in the United States due to prescription opioid overdose rose to more than fifteen thousand in 2015, according to the Centers for Disease Control.[31] Moreover, when people who are addicted to prescription opioids can no longer get them or need something stronger, many turn to heroin. One sad, high-profile case is the death of actor Philip Seymour Hoffman, who battled with prescription opioid addiction before dying of a heroin overdose at age 48.[32] Deaths from heroin overdose rose to thirteen thousand in 2015, higher than the number from gun-related homicides.[33]

Physicians as a group believe they are in part responsible for causing the opioid epidemic and now they are addressing it. In 2016, the American Medical Association, which has more than two hundred thousand physician members, recommended that pain should no longer qualify as the fifth vital sign. Proponents of removing pain as the fifth vital sign say that unlike all the other vital signs, which can be measured in objective terms, pain is subjective. One person's 10 can be another person's 4.

What does this mean for orthopedic patients? First, it means that orthopedic surgeons are also trying to do their part to decrease opioid use. Second, most orthopedic surgeons still use opioids, if more sparingly, because the majority of patients need them, at least for a short period of time. It is difficult for surgeons to avoid prescribing them.

The problems I observed occurred when patients took significant amounts of opioids before surgery and subsequently required increasingly higher levels to cover their pain. These patients were often miserable. As noted earlier, members of the medical profession are not going to pass judgment, but they can't help what they don't know. To avoid the risk of an overdose, please be forthright about opiate use prior to surgery.

THE MULTIMODAL APPROACH TO PAIN

There is not one perfect pain regimen that works for everybody. Each diagnosis is also different, as is each surgeon's strategy to address pain. The best advice is to communicate with your surgeon ahead of admission.

Here are some key tips about what types of drugs are commonly used in joint surgeries. One buzz phrase you may hear: surgeons are using a "multimodal approach" to pain.[34] This simply means they use various methods and combinations of drugs to target different pain pathways in the body, including injections, acetaminophen, nonsteroidal anti-inflammatories, opiates, and ice. To make it easier to understand, I will discuss the most commonly used drugs below, divided by category.

Regional Anesthetic, or Peripheral Nerve Block

A nerve block works to deaden the sensation that is controlled by the targeted nerve. A femoral nerve block, for instance, numbs the area on the front of the knee, where the nerve's distribution includes the region of the quadriceps muscles. Since the femoral nerve does not cover the hamstrings on the back of the knee—those muscles are controlled by the sciatic nerve—patients with femoral nerve blocks often ask why they have pain on the back of their knee, but none on the front.

Femoral nerve blocks were controversial in my hospital because they worked so powerfully that they not only numbed the sensory part of the nerve's distribution, but also temporarily blocked the motor part, for as long as twelve hours. This left the quadriceps muscles, which are essential to walking, nonfunctional. Consequently, many of our patients' surgical knees would collapse underneath them when they tried to walk while the block was still active. We tried applying temporary knee braces to patients with a femoral nerve block their first day after surgery, but these only provided adequate support about half of the time; we were often catching people by their gait belts as their surgical knee gave way inside the brace. When patients couldn't step fully on their new knee, they became frightened and confused, because they had been told they would be able to put full weight on it.

Another issue my therapy colleagues and I noted is that, in spite of strongly worded advice from physicians and nurses to take oral pain medications, people who received femoral nerve blocks often refused to start taking them because they were still numb from the nerve blocks.

"This is a piece of cake," they would say with false euphoria, not comprehending or believing that their pain would increase dramatically and suddenly when the block wore off. When this happened, many of these patients would be brought to tears by the fast onset of high levels of pain. If you do have a nerve block of any kind, please listen to your orthopedic nurse and start taking oral pain medications when you are advised to do so, so that the pain meds have time to take effect before your block runs out.

OrthoColorado no longer uses a femoral nerve block, having turned instead to an adductor-canal block, which relieves knee pain but does not affect the quadriceps function. Patients can walk safely with this block. However, many hospitals still use femoral nerve blocks.

If you have spine fusion or total ankle surgery, you may receive a sciatic block to numb the lower part of your body for a specific amount of time. Regional anesthetics are not typically used in total hip patients, as they are unnecessary.

Total shoulder patients are fortunate in that they can receive an interscalene block that paralyzes the shoulder during surgery, along with a numbing medication injected into the shoulder capsule at the end of surgery, so that their pain is addressed for 18 to 24 hours, but they can still move the hand.

Intra-articular Injections during Surgery

Some knee surgeons have moved away from nerve blocks altogether and have turned instead to local intra-articular injections, meaning injections of a numbing medication inside the joint. Rather than targeting a specific nerve's distribution, these injections work on smaller areas.

Drugs belonging to this category include lidocaine, bupivacaine, and ropivacaine. They work much like the novocaine you receive at the dentist's prior to having a cavity filled. These drugs can last anywhere from 8 to 36 hours. They are highly effective, and they also are highly local, so that when used in knee and hip patients, they do not prevent the person from walking safely. They also wear off more gradually than a nerve block.

Opioids

Opioids work by attaching to opioid receptors in your brain, spinal cord, and gastrointestinal tract, thereby blocking the pain messages your body is sending to your brain. Like your body's own endorphins, opioid drugs also prompt the nerve cells (neurons) to release dopamine, which is responsible for the euphoric "opioid effect." Because opioids are so effective, the right amount can allow you to participate in physical therapy and engage in other activities without undue pain. But opioids have side effects, as mentioned previously, including nausea, constipation, drowsiness, dizziness, and itching. They can also cause confusion and hallucinations. Patients over the age of 70 are at greater risk of these cognitive side effects because older people take longer to metabolize drugs.

While not widely utilized at my hospital, some surgeons still use a medication pump containing opioids, called a Patient-Controlled Analgesia pump, or PCA, which allows you to push a button when you need a dose of pain medicine. It is very important that you are the only person who pushes the pain button; family members should not push it while you are asleep, even if you appear to be in discomfort.

One of the most common questions patients ask is, "what's the difference between OxyContin and oxycodone?" OxyContin is a long-acting, time-release drug, which comes in different doses. It is usually given every 12 hours, in the morning and at night. You can remember it by thinking of "contin" as continuous. Another long-acting drug that is similar to Oxy-Contin is MS Contin, a type of morphine.

Oxycodone is the only ingredient in OxyContin, but oxycodone (another version is called Percolone) is a weaker dose and is given every 4 to 6 hours. Also, it is often combined with another drug, such as acetaminophen, commonly known as Tylenol. A Percocet 5/325, for instance, contains 5 mg of oxycodone and 325 mg of acetaminophen. Percocet can also come in other strengths, such as 7.5/325.

Another opiate you have likely heard of is Vicodin, which contains a narcotic called hydrocodone, plus 325 mg of acetaminophen. Vicodin also comes in different strengths, such as 5 mg, 7.5 mg, or 10 mg of hydrocodone. Other forms of hydrocodone with acetaminophen are Norco and Lortab.

And if you have heard of Dilaudid, the narcotic ingredient in it is called hydromorphone. It is given to people who can't tolerate oxycodone or hydrocodone, and it can be administered orally or via IV. It is also available in different dosages and is a short-acting medication.

Tramadol—or brand name Ultram—is a slightly less powerful synthetic opiate which also works on the brain to interfere with the perception of pain. Additionally, it functions like an antidepressant to increase the effects of serotonin and norepinephrine in the bloodstream. Tramadol is a less potent drug than hydrocodone or oxycodone, and it belongs to a less restrictive category, but it can be highly effective for moderate to severe pain. It can also help some patients who may not tolerate oxycodone, hydrocodone, or hydromorphone. Before you take tramadol, be sure to inform your physician if you are taking an antidepressant, as the two kinds of drugs can amplify each other and cause a dangerous hyper-stimulating effect.

Acetaminophen

Acetaminophen's brand names include Tylenol, Apap, and Anacin. Acetaminophen is a less potent pain reliever by itself, but its addition to hydrocodone to make Vicodin or oxycodone to make Percocet makes these drugs easier for the body to absorb. Acetaminophen can lower fever, reduce pain, and relieve headaches and minor aches. Unlike the next category, Nonsteroidal Anti-inflammatories (NSAIDs), acetaminophen does not reduce inflammation. It will not address swelling after orthopedic surgery.

Acetaminophen can also be given through an IV—this drug is called Ofirmev—and is effective in reducing moderate postoperative pain. Acetaminophen does not cause drowsiness.

Nonsteroidal Anti-inflammatory Drugs (NSAIDs)

Well-known NSAIDs include ibuprofen (Motrin, Advil), naproxen sodium (Aleve, Naprosyn), nabumetone (Relafen), indomethacin (Indocin), and aspirin. These drugs are mild pain relievers in small dosages and moderate pain relievers in higher dosages. They work by blocking the production of hormones called prostaglandins, which are produced by enzymes called

Cox-1 and Cox-2. Prostaglandins flood tissues that have been injured, for example by surgery, causing inflammation and sending pain signals to the brain. NSAIDs are effective at reducing inflammation, pain, and fever, but high dosages carry the risk of damaging the stomach lining. It is likely you will be asked to stop taking NSAIDs before surgery because of their blood-thinning effect and the potential risk of increased bleeding. However, in most cases you will be allowed to continue taking acetaminophen up until surgery.

Ketorolac, also known as Toradol, is a strong prescription NSAID given as a single injection or through the IV to significantly reduce pain caused by inflammation. It is powerful like an opioid but does not cause drowsiness. Ketorolac works well in post-op total knee patients to block the effects of prostaglandins, but because of its potentially serious side effects, including stomach bleeding and heart problems, it can only be given in limited doses and only to certain patients.

Celecoxib, also known as Celebrex, is the only drug of its kind approved by the FDA. As a Cox-2 inhibitor, celecoxib blocks the Cox-2 enzyme from making prostaglandin in parts of the body where inflammation is common, such as the joints. Unlike the other NSAIDs, which are both Cox-1 and Cox-2 inhibitors, celecoxib does not block prostaglandin from forming in the stomach, where the prostaglandin actually has a protective effect on the stomach lining. Celecoxib may be safer to use for people who suffer stomach distress or who are more susceptible to an ulcer in the intestines or the stomach. A similar drug, with a formula that is more than 90 percent a Cox-2 inhibitor, is meloxicam, with a brand name of Mobic.

Additional Medications

Some orthopedic surgeons may also prescribe medication to relieve nerve pain. Two of the commonly used drugs, especially for knee and spine patients, are gabapentin (Neurontin) and pregabalin (Lyrica). Both drugs are used to treat seizures and the pain of diabetic neuropathy and shingles.[35] Lyrica, a newer drug that is also used to treat fibromyalgia, can be given in smaller doses. These drugs may help to lower the use of opioids.

As noted, a multimodal approach to pain involves the use of different drugs and modalities such as ice and repositioning to reduce the perception of pain via different physiological pathways. In the multimodal approach, your pain regime could include one or more drugs from each of the above categories.

It is extremely important that you communicate to your surgeon, anesthesiologist, hospitalist, physician assistant, and nurse about any allergies or adverse effects you had from taking any of these drugs previously. One thing you should always do is take all pain meds with food. Some drugs may be off limits for people with a history of certain medical conditions, such as ulcers, stroke, or internal bleeding. The other thing to understand is that achieving pain relief without unpleasant side effects such as nausea and vomiting can take some trial and error, especially if you don't have a history of using these drugs. If you know that Percocet works for you, for example, but it makes you nauseous, you can be given an antiemetic scopolamine patch before surgery—but be sure to communicate your prior experiences with the anesthesiologist—as well as a number of other drugs to combat nausea afterward.

One commonly used drug to address nausea is Zofran, a very effective drug for some people. If you actually start vomiting, the drug of choice is Phenergan, but it causes drowsiness. When taking narcotics, you will also be given stool softeners, unless you have an inflammatory bowel disease. The best approach is to communicate regularly and clearly with your nurse about how you feel. The goal during the day should not be to put yourself into a state of stupor, but to find adequate pain relief without undue stomach upset, so that you can participate in physical therapy and other tasks that require moving, such as getting up to use the bathroom.

Chapter 8

Rehab Starts Now

I have a vivid memory of my mother after she had her knee replaced at the Hospital for Special Surgery (HSS) in New York City, where the first successful knee replacements were performed in 1974.

It was the early 1980s, and Mom was sitting on top of the kitchen table in our home in Connecticut, with her long legs hanging over the edge. She was bending her surgical knee as much as she could, and grimacing. It didn't look fun, but she kept going, using her good foot to pull the surgical-side foot further under the table to increase the bend.

"This is part of my home exercise program," she explained, gritting through her reps. "I need to get my knee bending as much as I can, but it hurts." Afterward, she sat in the living room with a big bag of ice on her knee and the leg elevated.

I didn't become a physical therapist until nearly twenty years later, but that image stuck with me because Mom was such a determined and conscientious patient. Later in life she was diagnosed with rheumatoid arthritis (in addition to osteoarthritis), which attacked multiple other joints in her body. Her hands and feet became deformed, the fingers and toes overlapping and contorting at unnatural angles. She had her second knee replaced, followed by her right shoulder in 1992. By the time her left shoulder needed replacement, she was too old. Her spine was also a mess, but she avoided back surgery and found relief with injections by a highly skilled physiatrist, a physician who treats pain by nonsurgical means. When Mom died at the age of 92, her knees had held up for thirty years and were the best joints in her body. She walked without knee pain, only using a cane or a walker when her back demanded it.

An otherwise healthy person, Mom spent at least a week in acute care at HSS for each surgery, and then another week or two in the rehab unit before she came home. Then she attended many weeks of outpatient therapy.

Mom was an orthopedic success story, especially given the deterioration of so many of her joints. These difficult but life-enhancing procedures allowed her to enjoy a high quality of life as long as she did.

Today, the surgical parts are much better—more anatomically designed, and made of stronger, lighter metals—and the recovery is a lot different. There is still a lot of rehab work to be done, especially for knee and shoulder patients, but much of that work today falls to you. Most patients today stay a night or two in the hospital and go directly home. Highly supervised rehabilitation for orthopedic patients is a thing of the past.

GETTING THE RIGHT THERAPY FOR YOU

No matter how you feel about the state of health care today, the good news is that total joint surgery today is highly successful. But it may come as a shock to learn that some total joint patients aren't getting any therapy at all. Pay attention, total hip patients: as health care dollars are stretched, it is no longer a given that you will receive the therapy services you may expect.

Rules have changed to save expensive spaces in rehab hospitals, where patients receive three hours of therapy daily, for those who have neurological accidents such as a stroke or spinal-cord injury or those suffering from a major trauma with multiple injuries. A knee replacement is not serious enough to automatically warrant a spot in a rehab facility, nor are any other joint replacement surgeries. Some patients who have bilateral knee replacement (both knees done in one operation under one anesthesia) may qualify for a rehab stay.

If you have a single joint surgery or a spinal fusion surgery you must demonstrate a need for skilled care to go to a skilled nursing facility (SNF, commonly known as a "Sniff.") In medical jargon, you have to "meet criteria," a phrase I heard frequently from a case manager when therapists would lobby for a patient to go to a skilled nursing facility out of concern for the patient's safety. Some patients had to pay privately for a SNF because they didn't have the benefit in their insurance plan or they didn't meet the criteria. The latter happened to people who lived alone and were highly functional and independent but declined to have anyone stay with them at home.

If you do go to a SNF, you should receive at least one hour a day of therapy, and your case manager should confirm this for you.

If you go directly home, you may receive home therapy two to three times weekly for two to three weeks if you have had a knee replacement. As someone who has worked in a hospital, an outpatient clinic, and in the home-care setting—and also as the spouse of a total knee patient—I firmly believe that the vast majority of total knee patients need home therapy. Most knee patients are better served in their own homes during the first two weeks, because the effort of getting dressed, getting in and out of the car—assuming someone can drive you—and traveling to an outpatient therapy appointment, is exhausting.

However, there is a growing trend to replace home physical therapy with outpatient physical therapy, at least for patients who have someone to drive them to the sessions. The reason is that outpatient PT is less expensive than home PT. While some patients may feel well enough to go directly to an outpatient clinic, many people, especially those over 65, prefer home PT. This decision should be based on what's best for you, not on the hospital's or the surgeon's agenda.

Shoulder, hip, ankle, and spine patients may receive no home therapy unless there is a safety concern. Shoulder, ankle, and spine patients usually go to outpatient therapy after a few weeks.

What does this mean for you? If you are a patient who expects physical therapy after a hip surgery, for example, you may not get any unless you ask for it. If you are committed to the best possible outcome—and you are if you are reading this book—you need to give this some thought, preferably ahead of surgery. Much of what happens in this regard depends on you—your interests and your activities. Are you satisfied to be able to walk a block in the community? Do you feel confident you can progress your own recovery safely, without supervision? Are you comfortable following a sheet of exercise instructions at home? If your answer to these questions is yes, you may do very well without outpatient therapy.

Or are you the person who expects to play golf or tennis or go downhill skiing in three months? Do you want to take long hikes and possibly summit a fourteen-thousand-foot peak? If you answer yes to these questions, you will want to pursue outpatient therapy. You will benefit from the expertise of a physical therapist to regain mobility, develop muscle strength, improve your balance, and address lingering tightness and pain.

Below are some general guidelines for what you may typically expect for each of the diagnoses covered, starting with therapy in the hospital and progressing through the outpatient experience. These are only guidelines.

TOTAL KNEE REPLACEMENT

A physical therapist will see you either the day of surgery or the morning after. You will also see an occupational therapist. The goals of these therapists are to make sure you will be safe to go home within your designated length of stay, usually a day or two. They will teach you how to get out of bed, which is called "bed mobility" in therapy terms. It is easier to move toward your nonoperative side. You will be taught safe "transfers," standing up from a bed or chair, and sitting down correctly, without plopping. This may sound easy but it is more difficult when one knee doesn't work yet and doubly difficult when both knees are replaced. You will need to show that you can walk household distances with a walker, crutches, or cane. And if you have stairs at home, either to get inside your home or to get to your bedroom, you will be taught, with assistance and a railing, how to negotiate them safely. Remember: up with the good leg, down with the surgical leg.

The occupational therapist needs to see that you can safely get in and out of a shower, or a tub with a shower, and on and off the toilet. The OT will also make sure you can dress yourself and provide tools to help you, unless you have a personal helper. If you were unable to perform these tasks before surgery, you will not be expected to perform them now without assistance, but the goal of therapy is to make you as independent as possible.

The PT will also teach you how to start moving your knee correctly and initiate the process of getting your range of motion back. You will learn some basic strengthening exercises, some strategies to keep your blood circulating and your swelling controlled, and best ways to position your knee for sitting and sleeping.

Once you are cleared by PT and OT to go home, and your medical status is stable, you will be discharged home with a loved one or caregiver (unless you go to a skilled nursing facility). Within one to two days your home physical therapy may begin. The home PT helps you through what can be a bumpy ride: while you need lots of rest, support, and basic care during these first few days at home, you also need to keep up with therapy, to prevent your knee from becoming too stiff. The home therapist gets you and your knee moving in a safe, supervised manner, pushing you enough so that you make progress and do things for yourself such as going up and down stairs.

Once you are able to get yourself dressed and out of the house and still have some energy left over, and perhaps even drive yourself, you will be transitioned to outpatient physical therapy. This could last anywhere from three to eight weeks, with one to three weekly sessions, depending on your needs and your insurance coverage. By the six-week mark, you should have excellent if not full range of motion in your surgical knee. Your bodily strength and overall endurance will begin to return. You may need a cane for longer walking distances. Outpatient therapy also addresses your quadriceps strength, and the strength of the surrounding muscles, as well as balance and coordination.

Throughout the rehab process you will develop a home exercise program, which you will want to maintain after the conclusion of PT. You will continue to make progress for anywhere from six months to two years. During this time, you may enjoy water therapy, such as walking against the current in an infinity pool.

If you go from the hospital to a skilled nursing facility (SNF), you should expect to stay for the minimum amount of time needed before you can take care of yourself at home. In the past, many patients stayed in a SNF for twenty-one days, because the SNFs stood to gain the best reimbursement from Medicare for this time frame. Needless to say, the time frame should be determined by your need, not the SNF's income. You may need five to ten days. When you leave, you may still expect to go to outpatient therapy.

HIP REPLACEMENT

The recovery from a routine hip replacement is generally easier and faster than for a routine knee replacement. Full recovery takes three to six months.

The hip is a ball-and-socket joint and second only to the shoulder as the most mobile joint in the body. Because of its structure, it moves in multiple planes and directions, whereas the knee is a hinge joint that moves primarily in one plane, like the elbow. Unlike the muscles and ligaments in the knee joint, which are configured to hold everything very snugly in place, those in the hip allow for a big range of movement. This means that getting your movement back after surgery is relatively easy if the implant fits well and the surgeon has done a good job.

The challenge lies in avoiding extremes of movement in the early stage of recovery that could cause the ball to slip out of the socket, which results in a painful dislocation. The movements you will need to avoid, if any, will depend on your surgeon's approach, whether posterior or anterior, and whether your surgeon believes precautions are necessary.

One of the first things your hospital PT and OT will ascertain when they see you, either the day of surgery or the morning after, is whether you understand your precautions if you have them and how they affect your daily function. If you are well prepared, you will know them and have considered how they will come into play at home. You will have thought about whether you need a raised toilet seat, or other adaptive equipment, as described in chapter 2. Depending on your precautions, you may need more occupational than physical therapy.

Both disciplines will teach you how to get out of bed correctly, which requires extra time and patience when you have hip precautions because of the prohibited movements. You will learn correct transfers and walking techniques. The PT will teach you how to negotiate stairs, and the OT will teach you how to shower, dress, and don and doff your socks and shoes. Even if you have no precautions, some of the movements required to dress your lower body may cause discomfort, so it is helpful to have a therapist teach you safe techniques. The OT will discuss a sock-aid and a long-handled shoehorn to allow you to perform these tasks independently. The OT will also teach you how to get in and out of a car. Hip patients generally need one to two days of therapy before they are cleared to go home.

In my orthopedic hospital, we taught our new hip patients the basic exercises described and illustrated in chapter 2. We also instructed them in more advanced sitting and standing exercises, sometimes in a group setting. Patients were then on their own to perform these advanced exercises until they returned to their surgeon's office about ten days later. Our hip patients did not routinely receive home physical or occupational therapy.

As noted above, outpatient therapy may not be automatically prescribed. If you think you would benefit from physical therapy, and especially if you wish to return to sports or physical activities, ask your surgeon for a prescription for a few outpatient PT visits.

SHOULDER REPLACEMENT

You will typically be seen by physical and occupational therapy in the hospital the morning after surgery. Depending on whether you had a traditional or reverse total shoulder, your therapists will reinforce the precautions your surgeon ordered, which consist of movements that could put your recovery at risk.

You will most likely have a sling or brace, and your OT will show you how to take it off and put it back on, with or without the assistance of your caregiver. You will take the brace off to shower and to perform your exercises. Otherwise, when you are sleeping or moving around, you will wear it to protect the delicate shoulder tissues as they heal.

Initially, the exercises will consist of moving the joints below the shoulder—bending and straightening your elbow, flexing and extending your wrist, and opening and closing your hand and fingers—to keep the blood flowing in the arm and to prevent stiffness. You will learn how to safely perform the pendulum exercise. One of your therapists may assess your walking safety; this is usually only an issue if you used an assistive device such as a walker or cane before surgery.

The OT will show you and your caregiver how to dress, eat, and bathe. You will need to perform personal hygiene with the nonoperative arm. Most total shoulder patients stay one to two nights before going home. You will continue with the home exercise program at home until you see your surgeon, who will give you a prescription to start outpatient physical therapy, typically at the two- to three-week mark.

You will see your outpatient therapist for eight to twelve weeks, approximately twice weekly. Your progress will depend in part on what condition your muscles and tendons were in prior to surgery, and how well your pain and swelling are managed. Each surgeon has a specific protocol for your therapist, and the first area of emphasis is to increase the mobility, or range of motion, in the shoulder. Your therapist will also teach gentle stabilization activities involving the shoulder blade and gentle isometric exercises (no movement, just tensing the muscles) to begin strengthening the muscles that have been immobilized in the sling.

At the six-week mark, you may have achieved about half of the full active range of motion of the arm, meaning you can move it in all directions on your own to half the extent that your other arm (or a normal arm) moves. And you can stop wearing the brace or sling. You will start to engage in more challenging strengthening exercises with the therapist's supervision.

Shoulder motion and strength should return to two-thirds of normal by the six-month mark and to full capacity by one year.

SPINE FUSION

Taking care of your neck and back is always important, but after a spine fusion surgery it becomes imperative. For an elegant short talk on why we need to take care of our back and our neck, watch two short videos by Princeton physician Grant Cooper on spine-health.com: "Why is Exercise Important for Low Back Pain?" and "Why is Exercise Important for Neck Pain?" Cooper explains the importance of strength for all of the back's structures, and the need for all the parts to work together in a coordinated manner. When one part weakens, the others compensate.

Once you have a fusion, the segments that have been fused together no longer move as two separate units. The parts of your back below and above the fused segments will start to compensate, by absorbing more of the forces of movement. In other words, the adjacent areas take up more work, and more stress. It is not uncommon for someone with a fusion at L4–L5, as an example, to need a second fusion later at L5–S1 or L3–L4. If you are a fusion patient who wants to maintain what you have and do everything you can to prevent another surgery, you need to accept an active role in caring for your neck and back for the rest of your life.

Whether your surgeon approached your spine from the front, the back, or the side, your therapy course after a fusion is the same. The goal of therapy is to ensure that you follow your spine precautions and that you move safely and correctly at a time when you are most vulnerable, as your tissues begin to heal.

Your first major task will be to master the log roll, as illustrated in chapter 2. It may be difficult and painful immediately after surgery, but it will become easier each time you do it.

If you have a lumbar fusion, your surgeon may order a back brace. You will learn how to put it on and take it off without twisting. You will practice safe transfers with good posture. Mostly, you will walk, initially with a walker to give you confidence and stability. Once you demonstrate that you consistently follow spine precautions and are able to walk safely and negotiate stairs, you will be discharged by your hospital PT.

Occupational therapy will also teach you how to dress, shower, and position yourself for sitting, sleeping, and everyday activities, with or without the use of devices such as a reacher, a sock aid, a long-handled shoehorn, and a long-handled sponge (for bathing).

When you leave the hospital, you should have a solid idea of what you need to do at home for the next six to twelve weeks until your outpatient therapy starts. In the initial stages of recovery, the most important thing is to allow the tissues to heal safely and the vertebrae to actually fuse together, without stress that would be caused by bending, lifting, or twisting. If you have a neck fusion, you may get a hard collar to protect and immobilize the area. But your lumbar spine doesn't get immobilized after an elective fusion; it relies on you to protect it by following your precautions (no bending, no lifting, no twisting; that is, no BLT).

However, it is also very important not to get any weaker by laying low and babying your neck or back out of fear of doing damage. Your spine heals best when you get serious about a walking program. Your initial starting point isn't as important as your new capacity to build endurance. A general goal spine surgeons will ask of you is to build up to walking two miles a day as soon as you are able, with pain being your guide. Stop and rest when you feel pain. If this distance is too much, start where you can and try to make regular progress. Your surgeon or hospital therapist can advise you individually.

Spine surgeons will order outpatient physical therapy between six and twelve weeks after your fusion, depending on how quickly you are healing. When you follow through with outpatient therapy, you will be taught additional activities and exercises to improve the strength throughout your core, legs, and back. How much therapy you need will depend again on you and your goals. Three months after surgery, a successful fusion should be set in place, and this is when many patients, especially those with a one-level fusion, are encouraged to increase activities that provide a positive stress to the bones in the spine. While further increases in core, leg, and back strength may continue to occur, a successful fusion is essentially healed at this time.

ANKLE REPLACEMENT

The biggest patient challenge for total ankle replacement patients is learning how to use a walker or crutches safely while not putting any weight on the surgical foot. Many of the postoperative ankle patients I worked with were advised preoperatively by their surgeon to acquire a device called a *knee walker*, an electric scooter with a resting platform for the surgical leg. This surgeon tells his patients that being non-weight bearing for six weeks is "not pleasant." I would add that if you get one, practice using it ahead of time for safe locomotion, especially on turns.

One brand of knee walker is the Roll-A-Bout, another is the KneeRover. The device resembles a scooter with two wheels in front and two in back that you propel with your good leg, while your surgical leg rests from the knee down on a padded surface that is parallel to the floor; the foot of that leg hangs off the back in a neutral non-weight-bearing position. These devices can handle ramps and can be broken down and transported in vehicles. However, they don't climb stairs. For that, you will either need to learn to use one crutch and a railing, or two crutches. And once you are upstairs, someone will have to carry it up for you. Some orthopedic practices rent knee walkers, or you can find a new or used one online. Insurance does not cover the cost.

Even if you get a knee walker, it is a good idea to learn how to take at least a few steps with crutches, which you will learn from your hospital physical therapist (or a pre-op PT consult). If you can't master crutches, you can try a walker for level surfaces. But if you have stairs at home and can't use crutches, you will need to learn how to "bump" up and down, which means sitting down with your back facing up the stairs and using your good leg to push yourself up, one step at a time. Once you get to the top, you will need to stand up and transfer to the knee walker.

Since the foot is at the bottom of the body, fluids tend to pool here, so it is very important in the first two weeks of healing to keep your lower leg elevated above the heart whenever you are not up and doing something. When you first leave the hospital, you will probably have a splint that can be loosened if swelling increases. After about two weeks, when the wound is healed, you will receive a boot to protect your ankle. You will also start outpatient physical therapy.

In outpatient therapy—typically ordered twice weekly for six weeks—you will begin to move the new joint in all directions. Since the leg has been immobilized and become weak, you will be given exercises to improve strength, not only in the ankle, but also the knee, hip, and core. Strengthening these larger muscle groups will help to reduce the stress you put on the new ankle joint. If you heal well, you may be allowed to get out of the boot and to bear weight on the foot after six weeks, but you may still need to wear a cast shoe, as your foot may be too swollen to fit into a regular shoe. A cast shoe has a sturdy sole with an open upper part made of canvas; the foot is held in place by Velcro straps across the top.[36]

Full recovery from an ankle replacement, including the ability to return to previously enjoyed sports, may take a year.

Chapter 9

The ABCs of Hospital Culture

If you haven't been in a hospital lately, you may be surprised at how much the culture of delivering care has changed. This is by and large a good thing. A buzzword in health care today is consumerism. Imagine you are a traveler staying in a reputable hotel. During and after your stay, you are encouraged to let others know, including the hotel ownership and the whole world reading reviews on the web, whether your expectations were met. What did you like about your experience? What should have been better?

This consumerist outlook is alive and well in hospitals, too. The hospital where you choose to have your surgery will likely solicit your feedback. Driving this new sense of accountability on the part of hospitals to consistently provide better service is a branch of the Department of Health and Human Services, the Centers for Medicare and Medicaid Services. Today, you are encouraged—and I suggest it is your responsibility, because you and all patients deserve the best care possible—to speak up during your hospital stay. The same applies after discharge, when you may be randomly asked to complete a survey with the bureaucratically unwieldy name of Hospital Consumer Assessment of Healthcare Providers and Systems, otherwise known as HCAHPS (pronounced H-Caps).[37]

The HCAHPS survey measures your degree of satisfaction with multiple providers in various categories. You are not required to complete it, but I highly encourage that you do, because it is your chance to vote and to contribute to making US hospitals more accountable for how you are treated. The key point here is that hospitals with unsatisfactory scores will have a percentage of their usual reimbursement for services withheld from Medicare, the primary insurer for Americans age 65 and older for inpatient hospital stays. You do not have to be a Medicare beneficiary, however, to receive or fill out the survey, which can be given by phone or in writing at any time from forty-eight hours to six weeks after your discharge. It cannot be given while you are still in the hospital.

The HCAHPS survey (see appendix) is not a perfect instrument, and it has met with considerable backlash.[38] But at the very least, what it has done so far is to encourage hospitals to conduct their own internal soul searching, to see what they are doing well and what needs to be improved. One of the biggest areas targeted for improvement in hospitals is how providers communicate with patients.

There is more to good communication than simply bedside manner. Your doctors, nurses, therapists, and all others are accountable to you for their decision making. They need to answer your questions thoroughly, and treat you with the respect you deserve. When they don't, you have the right to call them out. If you don't get your pain medication on time, you deserve an explanation. If you call for help to walk to the bathroom, and your nursing assistant or nurse doesn't come within a few minutes, you can expect to hear the reason. If a therapist makes an appointment to come at 2:00 p.m. and doesn't come until 2:30 p.m., you have a right to ask why. If a doctor comes and speaks with you, and afterward you have no idea who that was—this happened many times when I was in a patient's room—there is something wrong with the doctor's presentation. He spoke too quickly and didn't take the time to explain his role. Now with the HCAHPS survey there is something you can do about it.

Additionally, the stereotype of the paternalistic doctor-knows-best attitude is falling by the wayside. Physicians and their support staff need to make a greater effort to be sure you understand what they recommend, and why. You have every right to ask why you are receiving a medication in the morning that you would normally take at night. You should also be informed of the pros and cons of a recommended treatment or medication, possible side effects, why you need it, and whether there is a suitable alternative.

If you are curious about the most common patient complaints, here is one list, in no particular order, courtesy of a survey conducted at Johns Hopkins and first published in the *U.S. News and World Report* patient advice blog:[39]

- Being awakened between 10:00 p.m. and 6:00 a.m. for vitals or a blood draw and consequently not getting quality sleep
- Noisy nurses' stations
- Having your belongings lost
- People coming in to your room without knocking
- Not having the whiteboard in your room updated
- Not updating you or your family promptly of changes in your condition
- A dirty room with unpleasant odors
- Providers that don't listen carefully and don't seem to care if you understand your treatment plan
- Not getting clear instructions about using your remote or ordering food
- Lack of a professional attitude by employees when they are not providing direct care, such as when they are on break

In the orthopedic setting, you should not have to suffer silently through any of these situations, except possibly the first one: being awakened for a blood draw and vital signs. The timing of the blood draw is unfortunate, but it stems from medical necessity. Your blood values, including your hematocrit and hemoglobin, and clotting factors, need to be watched closely for any critical changes as a result of surgery. You have the right to ask why you need to be awakened and to ask why it is necessary to do the blood draw at that time. If you are told, "because the doctor ordered it," which doesn't give you a real reason, speak to the doctor or hospitalist. If you are courteous rather than accusatory, you should receive an answer that you fully understand.

All of the other complaints, should you find yourself in a situation to make them, are worthy and deserving of your critical and constructive feedback. These are things that shouldn't happen, but they do. As a clinician, one of my pet peeves was encountering whiteboards that weren't updated or even filled in. If a patient was experiencing significant pain, I wanted to know the timing and dosage of the most recent pain meds, so that I could assess whether there was something I could do to help, or whether I needed to wait and return later. Or I would look for the patient's weight bearing status, and it was missing, which meant that the aide coming in on the next shift to take the patient to the bathroom wouldn't know that he or she couldn't put any weight on the surgical ankle. My advice is if your floor nurse doesn't fill in your whiteboard when you are getting acquainted for the first time, ask that it be done and regularly updated. An up-to-date whiteboard will also help inform family members who come to visit, because you may be too sleepy or spacey to remember when you last had pain meds.

HOSPITAL ETIQUETTE IS A TWO-WAY STREET

Rest assured that most nurses and other clinicians have been grilled about appropriate and inappropriate behaviors toward patients. But what about *your* behavior toward them? How should you relate to them during your experience? What are your responsibilities?

Just as you would research and ask questions about a new car or any new product you plan to buy, you as the consumer also need to take responsibility for asking questions, speaking up, reporting your symptoms, and communicating with each of your providers. The best way you can help in the hospital is to communicate your needs clearly and politely, and expect to do so each time you see another clinician. Try to think of yourself as the key player in a team effort. Everyone on your team is rallying behind you, sometimes behind the scenes.

If you have a visitor when a provider comes to see you, consider whether you want your health-care information discussed in front of everyone in the room. If not, it is your responsibility to speak up and ask the visitors to leave. It is fine with most providers if one or two family members or close friends are present, as long as you can give your full-fledged attention to the task at hand. Phone conversations should be taken outside of the room. Loud dialogue between visitors in the room is disruptive. Children climbing on your bed or running around the room may be cute, but they make meaningful communication a challenge. Don't be surprised in this case if a physician or other provider asks your guests to step out of the room.

On the other hand, if the visitor is your basic support person, every provider should respect and appreciate his or her presence, unless the person is uncooperative or trying to answer questions directed specifically to you. In fact, both physical and occupational therapists will often set up a dedicated appointment for a "family training" session with your caregiver and you. Examples include a session with your caregiver and an occupational therapist if you are a total or reverse total shoulder patient who needs assistance getting dressed and taking your sling off and putting it back on; or a stair-training session with a physical therapist to teach your caregiver where to stand and how to guard you when you are negotiating stairs. Most providers like to see visitors, but not too many and not in a continuous stream that keeps you from getting much needed rest.

What about refusing care? It is your right to do so, but it is also your responsibility to provide a reason. If you are a Jehovah's Witness and do not wish to have a blood transfusion under any circumstances, it is in your best interests to make this known before your hospital admission. If you refuse physical or occupational therapy, there should be a good reason, such as vomiting, lightheadedness, or poorly controlled pain. If you refuse repeatedly, without apparent reason, as a small number of people do, you may be destined to go to a skilled nursing facility. There is no financial incentive to refuse therapy. You are not charged for each therapy session, even if you do see a line item on your bill. Charges for therapy are included in the lump sum that is contracted between the hospital and your insurance; the same is true if you have arranged to pay out of pocket. Refusing therapy for unjustified reasons tends to backfire, as it is putting off the inevitable. Providers know you are likely exhausted and possibly hurting. If you ask your therapist in the morning to please give you time to nap between 2:00 p.m. and 3:00 p.m., for example, this can usually be accommodated. Don't be afraid to ask for a specific appointment time if you wish.

The majority of patients I worked with were cooperative and respectful. Most were receptive, and they understood that I was there to help, not hurt them, even though therapy does sometimes hurt. Other patients didn't follow the advice of doctors, nurses, and therapists, who have seen hundreds or thousands of others in the same predicament. Here's a simple cardinal rule of behavior: do what your providers tell you to do. They actually do know better. If you object or don't understand, ask why the advice is important. If a nurse advises you to eat crackers or other food with your pain meds, it is to ward off nausea. If a therapist tells you to stay up for just one to two hours in a chair after therapy and then call your nurse or aide to help you back to bed, it is to conserve energy so you can get up again later.

One morning at 10:00 a.m., an occupational therapist and I assisted a knee replacement patient out of bed and to a chair. She had not attended our preoperative education class. We explained that the reason her knee was buckling was because she had a nerve block, which was also why she wasn't feeling much pain. We knew the block would wear off by the afternoon. We assisted her to her recliner and told her to stay up for one to two hours—no longer—then call her CNA to help her back to bed, where her knee would be iced and elevated. I told her I would return in the afternoon once the block had worn off to see if she could take a walk.

When I returned four hours later, she was just going back to bed with the CNA.

"There's no way I can get up again now," she complained tearfully. "I'm just getting back to bed."

The CNA had tried to persuade her to go back to bed at noon, but the patient refused because her son was visiting. At 4:30 p.m., after my shift had ended, I was still in the building and received a call that the patient's daughter was visiting now and was angry that the patient hadn't received her second therapy visit (although it had been refused.) I stayed to work with her. The CNA and I assisted her to the bathroom, and all she could do afterward was walk from the toilet to the chair. She cried throughout the session. She hadn't followed basic instructions and was suffering the consequences.

This scenario played out over and over again. Sometimes patients don't trust their CNA or their nurse to get them back to bed, so they stay up until the therapist returns. Then they are too tired to participate in therapy, and all they want to do is go back to bed.

If you are told to use your oxygen while sleeping, or to drink more fluids, but you aren't sure why these things matter, please ask. If you are told "to call, not fall," it means just that, because a fall could mean another trip to the operating room. Do not try to get up on your own; you could pull out your IV or trip over a line that hasn't been detached. Do not ask your family member to take you to the bathroom or assist you back to bed unless a therapist has trained that person and has written on your whiteboard that it is okay.

I once had an elderly spine patient who was weak and woozy when we worked with her. She had not attended spine class, she said, because her partner was a nurse and knew all about these things. But the partner had never worked as an orthopedic nurse and had retired from nursing years earlier. Neither of them had any knowledge of the log roll technique. The OT and I instructed her in the log roll, but she needed a lot of coaching and hands-on help. We told her that she must call when she wanted to move back to bed and not try to get up by herself or with her partner, who had not yet arrived.

Thus, we were both worried to learn later that afternoon that when the partner arrived, the patient had gone back to bed without calling, and later got up and went for a walk with the partner. The patient claimed not to have remembered our warning, which we had written on the whiteboard. The partner, who was not very mobile herself, had pulled the patient up from the chair incorrectly, stressing the spinal structures. We don't know how she helped the patient back to bed and back out again. We had a heart-to-heart with the patient and the partner, who protested that she was a nurse and knew what she was doing. We also spoke with the patient's nurse, who was new and needed more education about safe spine techniques.

Always ask if you don't understand an instruction or why it is necessary to follow certain rules. The grand mission of the entire staff is to keep you safe, and as comfortable as possible, and you are the centerpiece of that mission.

The take-home message is that hospital etiquette is a two-way street. Nurses in particular get stressed and overextended, and you can influence how they care for you by simply acting civil. Try to consolidate your requests for things, so that people aren't running back and forth to get water, then coffee, then ice, then a drink for your visitor, for example. By treating your caregivers as trained professionals, and by following the golden rule of treating others as you would like to be treated, you will receive care in a kinder and more nurturing manner in return.

Chapter 10

Homeward Bound

The following is not a happy story, but I am sharing it so you can avoid a similar experience.

My friend Ann went to an out-of-state orthopedic specialty hospital for her total knee replacement. She had an uneventful hospital course and was discharged home at 1:00 p.m. on a Friday after a two-night stay. Her next dose of pain medication was due at 3:30 p.m. Her husband drove her home, got her settled, and went to a nearby pharmacy to fill her prescription.

Her insurance refused to cover the prescription for oxycodone, because the amount prescribed was more than her policy covered. Many phone calls and hours later, a nurse at her surgeon's office was able to solve the problem—the number of pills was reduced—and Ann finally received her first dose of pain medicine, ninety minutes late. The experience was frightening and exhausting, not how she wanted her return home to begin.

Her saga didn't end there. Her home physical therapist, the only clinician who saw her for two weeks, was concerned because Ann was wheezing and had a rash with hives, likely caused by the oxycodone. She had received prescription-strength Benadryl in the hospital, but neither she nor her husband "remembered anyone ever talking to us at the discharge about the side effects [of opioids]," and no prescription was written to address them at home.

Another round of phone calls later, the surgeon's office switched her pain medication first to hydrocodone (Vicodin), which she vomited up immediately, and then to hydromorphone (Dilaudid), but the instructions were written incorrectly, telling her to take only half as much as she actually needed.

Unfortunately, this type of problem happens too frequently, because neither physicians nor patients know in advance what insurance will cover. Ann's primary-care physician, who was more accessible, came to the rescue by giving her a prescription for Tylenol with codeine, which she had taken and tolerated before.

Ann finally saw her surgeon at a six-week follow-up visit, having seen the PA at an earlier visit because the surgeon was on vacation. But when she told the doctor an abbreviated version of what had happened with her medications, instead of listening he "cut to the chase. All he wanted to know was which drug I had taken the most."

"This man is a wonderful surgeon, but his practice is too big," she says. "You cannot talk to anybody."

Multiple mistakes were made, and the surgeon's office failed to acknowledge the existence of a problem, much less apologize. The errors will likely occur again. When you meet with your surgeon preoperatively, ask about the flow of communication and specifically how you will be able to reach him. Some surgeons give patients their cell phone number.

Fortunately, Ann progressed in outpatient PT and stopped taking pain medication except for one Tylenol with codeine at night by the eight-week mark. She is grateful to her primary care physician for rescuing her during the medication crisis. Her advice to others: be as aware as you can, and be proactive. Having an informed partner close by helps, because "you are really out of it for a week after surgery."

TAKE YOUR DISCHARGE SERIOUSLY

Your discharge from the hospital is an extremely important transition. Yet when it is your time to leave, you may be drug-addled and sleep-deprived. Some if not most of the material the nurses, doctors, and therapists tell you will sail over your head. So the number one recommendation is to not go through this alone. Your caregiver needs to be by your side.

Don't ask your caregiver to come pick you up at the last minute. Both of you should know the approximate time of your discharge at least the day before, whether it is targeted for the morning or the afternoon. Again, do not even try to go through the motions of getting discharged until your caregiver arrives.

Besides being cleared by therapy, here are a few basic medical criteria that should be met before you are discharged. You should be holding down food. You should be urinating on your own and have active bowel sounds. You should not have a fever, and your pain should have been managed for the past twelve hours without the need for IV pain medications. Assuming these criteria have been met, here are the key things that will be covered at the discharge. Before you and your caregiver nod in agreement and allow your nurse to rush to the next item, be sure to get your questions answered.

Concerns

Two of the most dangerous complications that can arise during recovery are wound infections and blood clots, known as deep vein thrombosis (DVT). It is important that you understand the signs and symptoms of each before being discharged.

An infected incision isn't just red and warm; nurses describe it as looking "angry." The difference may be hard to discern to the uninitiated, but a certain amount of redness around your incision is normal. Ask your nurse to discuss this with you at your discharge.

Likewise, the symptoms of a blood clot are sometimes difficult to differentiate from normal swelling after surgery. Signs of a blood clot are calf pain or nonincisional leg pain, redness around the knee, and excessive swelling in any part of the leg. Be sure you tell your medical team if you have ever had a blood clot before. About 1 in 100 knee patients and 1 in 200 hip patients contract a blood clot regardless of the multifaceted efforts to prevent one (including the compression pumps, the ankle pump exercise, early walking, and the administration of blood-thinning medication). If a clot is found in the hospital, by means of an ultrasound image, it can be treated with extra blood-thinning medication. A blood clot that travels to your lungs, called a pulmonary embolism, is a potentially life-threatening emergency. Your nurse should educate you about the symptoms of a blood clot and a pulmonary embolism. Symptoms of the latter include chest pain, shortness of breath, anxiety, and a dry cough. If you suspect a blood clot or a pulmonary embolism, you will be instructed to call the hospital or 911.

Ask your nurse what to do if you contract a fever. A fever of 100 degrees two days after surgery, which my husband had, probably does not mean you have a wound infection, but rather that you are fighting an excess of fluid in your lungs. A post-surgical fever of 101.5 degrees that lasts more than twenty-four hours warrants a call.

Medications

You will receive a list of your current medications. Be sure the list includes any drugs you were taking before surgery, especially those you take on a regular basis, such as thyroid or cholesterol or blood pressure medication. Be sure you understand the dosage of blood thinner you are receiving, how long you are supposed to take it, and whether it interferes with any of the other medications on your list. Your nurse should be on top of this.

You may not be allowed to take nonsteroidal anti-inflammatories (NSAIDs) for a certain period of time while also taking blood thinners. However, if you only take aspirin as a blood thinner, you may be allowed to take celecoxib or meloxicam. There are exceptions to every rule, but it is best to ask.

It is important to know that you should not take more than 3 grams of acetaminophen (the ingredient in Tylenol) in a 24-hour period; the former daily limit was 4 grams. Some narcotic medicines also contain acetaminophen, such as 325 mg in a single Norco or Vicodin. If any clinician advises you to take more acetaminophen for breakthrough pain, that person should first know how much you are already taking. You can protect yourself by keeping track of the total amount you take daily. Taking too much can cause irreversible kidney and liver damage.

If you take vitamins or any natural remedies at home, be sure to ask your nurse if and when it is okay to resume taking these.

The list of medications should not include any new ones containing ingredients that have caused an allergic reaction in the past.

Know the side effects of each new medication. Does it cause a rash? What kind of adverse reaction, such as wheezing, should concern you? Do you have something to take for nausea and for constipation?

If possible, get your first prescription for pain medication filled while you are still at the hospital. If the hospital does not have a pharmacy, ask your caregiver to fill it nearby before you leave. The nursing staff will have a list of nearby pharmacies.

Understand what your caregiver needs to do to get a refill of any medication, especially a narcotic. This cannot be called in by a doctor's office; someone will need to pick up a written prescription for you. Whom will you call when you need a refill? Get a contact number, ideally at your surgeon's office, that allows you to reach someone on call 24/7. You will have to wait for a call back, but it shouldn't take all day. Don't let your medications run out before you know how you will get the next prescription.

Ask your PA or your nurse when and how to wean yourself off your narcotic pain medications. Don't keep taking them just because you have them; if your pain levels are improving on a daily basis you don't need as much. Weaning off these medications should not require guesswork, but in my experience patients are rarely told how to do it.

When my husband had his knee replaced, the surgeon generously and routinely gave his cell phone number to his post-op patients. Just having it was a source of comfort to us. The first time I called because Ernie had a fever and uncontrollable shakes the night he came home. His doctor reassured me that nothing was seriously wrong, in part because his fever was only 100 degrees. I heated a few blankets in the dryer, a trick I learned at the hospital, and they completely saved the day. His symptoms resolved.

The second time I called, it was to find out which pain medication to cut back on first (when he felt ready), and how then to handle the breakthrough pain. Even as a hospital PT with a respectable foundation in pharmaceuticals, I was uncertain how best to reduce his narcotics without professional advice. Ask your PA and your nurse how to handle your specific regimen.

Don't be afraid or bashful to ask questions before you leave, while you still have a live audience. And if you get a precious moment with your surgeon, ask if you could have his cell phone number, just to alleviate your anxiety. What do you have to lose? It's not an unreasonable request.

Equipment

Before you leave, you should either be in possession of the equipment you will need or else know how you are getting it. You can usually get a walker, cane, and crutches through the hospital's therapy department, and there shouldn't be any markup in price. Even the hospital gift shop should have good prices for other items you may need. At our hospital, if we didn't have the available equipment, we had a list of nearby vendors who would deliver what you needed to your hospital room.

Follow-Up Appointments

If you don't already have an appointment to see your surgeon (or the PA), find out when to go, and make this appointment soon. A common interval is ten days to two weeks after surgery. In the meantime, to reiterate, get at least one good contact number to call (if not your surgeon's), preferably of someone who has met you. You will likely run out of pain medications before your follow-up appointment.

Make sure you understand whether you need to see your primary care physician for any reason, such as a blood draw. Also, find out if you need to take a prophylactic antibiotic when you see the dentist. The reason for this is that when your mouth bleeds, which is a common occurrence during dental procedures, bacteria there can travel through your bloodstream to the surgical area and cause an infection.

Do you know when to expect to be contacted by a home health agency or the specific home therapist? If you are a knee patient who is going to outpatient therapy in a day or two, have you scheduled a few appointments in advance? This is something you should do before admission, even if you have to cancel with a 24-hour notice, because there may be a wait of a week or two to get an appointment.

Going for More Rehab

If you are going to a skilled nursing facility (SNF), a lot of things should be taken care of for you, including the transfer of all your medications from the hospital to the new destination.

But there are a few basic things you might want to know. Will you have a private room? How long are you projected to stay, and who determines the schedule? Who will be responsible for your medical care when you go to the SNF? How much therapy will you receive there? If you have other scheduled medical appointments, will you be able to keep them and will you be transported? Lastly, is there someone in your hospital you can contact in the event of a problem with your care at the SNF?

A tip: it is customary for the last facility where you stay to issue equipment for home use. So if you are going from the hospital to the SNF, don't worry about taking a walker—the SNF will provide one as needed.

Activities

If you go to a SNF, your schedule will be structured around meal times and therapy sessions. If you go home, you will have control over how you spend your time. Find out if there are any activities you should avoid during the first week or two until you see your surgeon. If there is a special event you want to attend, especially if it involves flying, ask if or when it is okay to do so.

Do you know your precautions? Are there specific exercises you should be doing, per physical or occupational therapy? Do you have written copies? Do you know how best to elevate and ice your surgery site?

When can you get your wound wet?

Are there any specific dietary recommendations?

Do you and your caregiver have an idea of how long you will need hands-on care and when it is okay to leave you alone for a few hours?

Finally, do you and your support team feel that your questions have been answered and that you know what to do when you go home?

Home at Last

On a short drive home, it's best not to stop any more than necessary. However, if you have a long ride—in Colorado, many of our patients traveled from out of state—be sure to plan regular breaks for getting out to stretch. Your occupational therapist can provide tips for making a long ride more comfortable. It is better to sit in the front seat than to lie down in the back.

Once you get home, your care doesn't simply end. You will still need consistent round-the-clock care, someone to watch over you, prepare at least some of your meals, take care of household chores, monitor your medications, and keep an eye on how you are doing. One friend of mine got a whiteboard for home use just for keeping track of her medications.

Your body will recover dramatically in the next few weeks, although you may not feel it immediately. It is best, unless a physician has instructed you otherwise, to get out of bed every day, get dressed, and sit at the table for meals. Try to find a routine that provides a healthy balance of moving and resting.

This is also a good time to relax and be kind to your body and your psyche. Carve out ample space and energy to devote to your home exercise program if you have one. Then take the time to elevate and ice your surgical site afterward. Walk around your home frequently, every waking hour if possible. Be sure to keep up with stool softeners if you are taking narcotics. Drink more water.

Healing is something you can't easily see, and it demands your utmost patience. While recovery times vary from diagnosis to diagnosis and from patient to patient, basic wound healing and healthy scar formation are natural biological processes that take a more-or-less fixed amount of time. It's not just the multiple layers of skin in the wound that need to heal. Layers of muscle have been stretched or cut and subsequently reattached. Sometimes, it seems that the youngest, fittest and most muscular people, whether male or female, struggle more with pain than thinner, older people. Muscle tissue has a healthy supply of blood vessels and nerve endings. Nerves allow us to feel, including pain. Remember, pain = healing.

DRIVING AND WORKING

Research shows that patients with a surgery on their right leg, including a knee, hip, or ankle replacement, need about one month to regain their ability to apply the brakes at a safe speed.[40] The speed of braking is just one important parameter to consider when resuming driving. If you are taking narcotics for pain, your reaction time will remain compromised. Surgeons differ on this issue, and of course the timing depends on whether your surgery is on the left or the right side. I would suggest asking your surgeon ahead of time, and this will help you plan your outpatient appointments as well.

Interestingly, the same study found that shoulder patients who wore a brace or a sling had impaired driving ability for a longer period than those who didn't. The average return to driving for total shoulder patients in this study was one to three months.

Spine fusion patients actually had normal brake times on average at the time of their hospital discharge, but most reported waiting six weeks before driving.

Other things to consider about driving, besides your doctor's recommendations, are the distance you need to travel, the amount of traffic, and the familiarity of the route. Most physicians I know tell their patients not to drive while still taking narcotics.

My advice is to be conservative and use caution. It might be okay to drive to your outpatient PT appointment just a short distance away, but not to drive in a city or on a highway or on multiple errands. Your best bet is to line up someone to drive you to your first few outpatient appointments.

Many patients ask when they can return to work. If you normally drive to work, your return will depend on when you can drive. If you work from home or are able to take public transportation, you may be able to resume part-time desk work after two to three weeks, but don't be surprised if sitting at a computer for several hours exhausts you. A more realistic return for someone with a desk job is six weeks after surgery. And if you have a job that requires physical work, it will take longer, about three months, but this depends on your specific surgery as well as the nature of your job.

SPORTS

You will be able to return to sports. In my active state of Colorado, it is common to see people skiing (downhill and cross-country), hiking, snowshoeing, playing doubles tennis, and golfing several months after their surgeries. Road biking is fine; mountain biking is okay as long as it's not too aggressive. Downhill mountain-bike racing would not be a good idea. Running long distances is generally ill-advised after a knee, ankle, or hip replacement, but swimming is recommended.

Hip and Knee Patients

Generally, hip and knee surgeons are becoming more liberal about allowing patients to return to sports. This is based in part on the improvement in the design of implants and the fact that they last longer.

Today, you have about a 90 percent chance that your total knee will last fifteen years, and an 85 percent chance it will last twenty years or more.[41] And for total hips, about 90 to 95 percent last ten years, while 80 to 85 percent last twenty years or more. Also, the plastic spacer component used in knee replacements is not terribly difficult to remove and replace if it wears out. However, if a metal component in any prosthesis is broken and more bone needs to be sacrificed to replace it, a revision surgery becomes more complicated and potentially less successful.

At the three-month mark, many surgeons will give you the green light to downhill ski, ice skate, bike, and play doubles tennis, especially if you have done these things previously with some proficiency. But it is risky to take up a new sport such as skiing or snowboarding after a knee or hip replacement, because beginners tend to fall frequently. While it's not likely you will loosen a well-placed prosthesis, you will subject it to greater wear and tear. Some doctors may advise against mogul skiing.

It is best to avoid sports and activities that put a tremendous amount of stress on these joints. Running triples the amount of force on the knees compared to walking. Sports like soccer, basketball, singles tennis, baseball, or squash and racquetball involve running and high impact, and these should be played in moderation or avoided. And while you can run short distances occasionally if it doesn't hurt, it's not the best time to run your first 10K or compete in the running portion of a triathlon (although the swimming and biking parts are fine).

It is important to have realistic expectations.

Golf is a safe bet, as are hiking, swimming, and rowing. Strengthening activities such as yoga and weightlifting are also good and recommended. As long as you don't repeatedly pound and twist your knee or hip, you should be able to do most of the things you did before.

As one surgeon I know likes to tell his patients: "This is not your knee when you were twenty."

Total Shoulder Patients

There is less research on returning to sports after a total shoulder replacement, but the outlook is positive. According to one review of the literature in the *World Journal of Orthopedics*, most shoulder surgeons now allow their patients to return to non-contact sports within six months after a total shoulder (TSA) or reverse total shoulder replacement (rTSA).[42] In this literature survey, more than 75 percent of all total shoulder patients reported returning to their previous sports.

A different study in the *American Journal of Sports Medicine* of patients with one or more total shoulder replacements showed that 71 percent who wanted to return to sports not only did so, but reported that their ability improved.[43] And half were able to play their sport more often. The most popular sports they participated in were swimming, golf, and tennis. Only 20 percent who wanted to return to softball were able to do so.

Some shoulder surgeons encourage patients to return to their sport if they have good general health and good activity levels before surgery.[44] They allow patients to return to activities like tennis, golf, fishing, swimming, and light weight lifting but discourage ultra-high-impact activities like boxing, shotgun shooting, or heavy powerlifting. They also discourage waterskiing and contact sports.

Spine Patients

If you are having a neck or back fusion surgery and would like to resume playing recreational sports such as golf or tennis, you will probably be able to do so. Much of the literature about cervical (neck) spine patients returning to sports focuses on professional athletes, including pro wrestlers, golfers, and football players. Peyton Manning is a famous example, as well as an exceptional one; he underwent an anterior cervical discectomy and fusion and later led the Denver Broncos to the 2016 Super Bowl victory.

The literature suggests that people who undergo a one-level fusion with an approach from the front, called an anterior cervical discectomy and fusion (ACDF), are able to return to most previous sports, with the exception of snowboarding.[45] However, most people with a high cervical fusion, at C1-2, will not be allowed to return to contact sports, because the risk of a devastating injury is too great.[46]

If you are a low-back patient and truly dedicated to a specific sport, be sure to discuss this with your surgeon before your operation. Generally, your chances of resuming a sport are better if you have a fusion of one or two levels as opposed to three or four. When the vertebrae that make up the bony spine are implanted with grafted bone and connected to one another with hardware, they need a significant amount of time to fuse together into a structural and functional unit. Subsequent to a fusion, the vertebrae above and below the now immobilized unit will absorb more of the impact of movement, whether bending, twisting, pounding, or sideways sheer force. The more units that are fused together, the stiffer and less mobile the spine becomes. In the case of a three- or four-level fusion, returning to a contact sport or a high-impact activity may be too risky.

But if you have a smaller fusion and you enjoyed a sport before surgery—and you work hard in physical therapy to strengthen your back, core, and legs—you may be able to return to your sport at the three to six-month mark. In one study of golfers with a one- or two-level lumbar fusion, more than half returned to playing on a golf course within the first year of surgery.[47] But, experts caution, you should be pain-free, have good sensation and muscle control—indicating that your nerves are fully intact—and have successfully completed a course of physical therapy. In the golf study, 29 percent of the patients reported that ongoing back and leg pain limited their ability to resume playing golf.

Ankle Patients
If you are a total ankle patient who likes to swim, cycle, or work out at the gym, you are in good company. In a study of 101 total ankle patients,

about two-thirds of them were active in a sport 3.7 years after surgery.[48] Two-thirds of the active patients said they were better at their sport after surgery.

FINAL THOUGHTS

When I taught the physical therapy portion of Joint Class to the prospective knee and hip replacement patients at my hospital, I always wished everyone good luck. As I stood there watching them file out of the room, I was confident that for virtually all of them it would be a positive change in their lives. After all, they had taken the initiative to learn about their various procedures, often bringing family members or caregivers along so they could be educated too.

That's how I feel about each of you who have read this book. I hope these chapters have assured you that these elective orthopedic surgeries have a high rate of success, and their whole purpose is to reduce pain and improve your quality of life.

And I hope you have a better understanding of your own role in this recovery, the part that Dr. Foran describes in the foreword as being 90 percent up to you. Remember, you are the most important player. You now know what you can do to prepare ahead of time, what to expect at the hospital, and how you and your caregivers can manage your recovery.

Whether you are committed to resuming a sport that you love, or simply want to go about daily life, walking your dog or visiting grandchildren, chances are very high that you will succeed.

Work hard, but work smart. Go for it, but not all at once. Be patient. Enjoy your new life. And good luck.

Appendix

HCAHPS Survey

HCAHPS Survey

SURVEY INSTRUCTIONS

♦ You should only fill out this survey if you were the patient during the hospital stay named in the cover letter. Do not fill out this survey if you were not the patient.

♦ Answer <u>all</u> the questions by checking the box to the left of your answer.

♦ You are sometimes told to skip over some questions in this survey. When this happens you will see an arrow with a note that tells you what question to answer next, like this:

    ☐ Yes
    ☑ No   ➔ *If No, Go to Question 1*

> *You may notice a number on the survey. This number is used to let us know if you returned your survey so we don't have to send you reminders.*
> *Please note: Questions 1-25 in this survey are part of a national initiative to measure the quality of care in hospitals. OMB #0938-0981*

Please answer the questions in this survey about your stay at the hospital named on the cover letter. Do not include any other hospital stays in your answers.

YOUR CARE FROM NURSES

1. **During this hospital stay, how often did nurses treat you with <u>courtesy and respect</u>?**
   - ¹☐ Never
   - ²☐ Sometimes
   - ³☐ Usually
   - ⁴☐ Always

2. **During this hospital stay, how often did nurses <u>listen carefully to you</u>?**
   - ¹☐ Never
   - ²☐ Sometimes
   - ³☐ Usually
   - ⁴☐ Always

3. **During this hospital stay, how often did nurses <u>explain things</u> in a way you could understand?**
   - ¹☐ Never
   - ²☐ Sometimes
   - ³☐ Usually
   - ⁴☐ Always

4. **During this hospital stay, after you pressed the call button, how often did you get help as soon as you wanted it?**
   - ¹☐ Never
   - ²☐ Sometimes
   - ³☐ Usually
   - ⁴☐ Always
   - ⁹☐ I never pressed the call button

YOUR CARE FROM DOCTORS

5. **During this hospital stay, how often did doctors treat you with <u>courtesy and respect</u>?**

   ¹☐ Never
   ²☐ Sometimes
   ³☐ Usually
   ⁴☐ Always

6. **During this hospital stay, how often did doctors <u>listen carefully to you</u>?**

   ¹☐ Never
   ²☐ Sometimes
   ³☐ Usually
   ⁴☐ Always

7. **During this hospital stay, how often did doctors <u>explain things</u> in a way you could understand?**

   ¹☐ Never
   ²☐ Sometimes
   ³☐ Usually
   ⁴☐ Always

THE HOSPITAL ENVIRONMENT

8. **During this hospital stay, how often were your room and bathroom kept clean?**

   ¹☐ Never
   ²☐ Sometimes
   ³☐ Usually
   ⁴☐ Always

9. **During this hospital stay, how often was the area around your room quiet at night?**

   ¹☐ Never
   ²☐ Sometimes
   ³☐ Usually
   ⁴☐ Always

YOUR EXPERIENCES IN THIS HOSPITAL

10. **During this hospital stay, did you need help from nurses or other hospital staff in getting to the bathroom or in using a bedpan?**

    ¹☐ Yes
    ²☐ No ➜ **If No, Go to Question 12**

11. **How often did you get help in getting to the bathroom or in using a bedpan as soon as you wanted?**

    ¹☐ Never
    ²☐ Sometimes
    ³☐ Usually
    ⁴☐ Always

12. **During this hospital stay, did you need medicine for pain?**

    ¹☐ Yes
    ²☐ No ➜ **If No, Go to Question 15**

13. **During this hospital stay, how often was your pain well controlled?**

    ¹☐ Never
    ²☐ Sometimes
    ³☐ Usually
    ⁴☐ Always

14. **During this hospital stay, how often did the hospital staff do everything they could to help you with your pain?**

    ¹☐ Never
    ²☐ Sometimes
    ³☐ Usually
    ⁴☐ Always

15. **During this hospital stay, were you given any medicine that you had not taken before?**

$^1\square$ Yes

$^2\square$ No ➔ **If No, Go to Question 18**

16. **Before giving you any new medicine, how often did hospital staff tell you what the medicine was for?**

$^1\square$ Never

$^2\square$ Sometimes

$^3\square$ Usually

$^4\square$ Always

17. **Before giving you any new medicine, how often did hospital staff describe possible side effects in a way you could understand?**

$^1\square$ Never

$^2\square$ Sometimes

$^3\square$ Usually

$^4\square$ Always

WHEN YOU LEFT THE HOSPITAL

18. **After you left the hospital, did you go directly to your own home, to someone else's home, or to another health facility?**

$^1\square$ Own home

$^2\square$ Someone else's home

$^3\square$ Another health facility ➔ **If Another, Go to Question 21**

19. **During this hospital stay, did doctors, nurses or other hospital staff talk with you about whether you would have the help you needed when you left the hospital?**

$^1\square$ Yes

$^2\square$ No

20. **During this hospital stay, did you get information in writing about what symptoms or health problems to look out for after you left the hospital?**

$^1\square$ Yes

$^2\square$ No

OVERALL RATING OF HOSPITAL

Please answer the following questions about your stay at the hospital named on the cover letter. Do not include any other hospital stays in your answers.

21. **Using any number from 0 to 10, where 0 is the worst hospital possible and 10 is the best hospital possible, what number would you use to rate this hospital during your stay?**

$^0\square$ 0   Worst hospital possible

$^1\square$ 1

$^2\square$ 2

$^3\square$ 3

$^4\square$ 4

$^5\square$ 5

$^6\square$ 6

$^7\square$ 7

$^8\square$ 8

$^9\square$ 9

$^{10}\square$ 10   Best hospital possible

22. **Would you recommend this hospital to your friends and family?**

   $^1\square$ Definitely no

   $^2\square$ Probably no

   $^3\square$ Probably yes

   $^4\square$ Definitely yes

UNDERSTANDING YOUR CARE WHEN YOU LEFT THE HOSPITAL

23. **During this hospital stay, staff took my preferences and those of my family or caregiver into account in deciding what my health care needs would be when I left.**

   $^1\square$ Strongly disagree

   $^2\square$ Disagree

   $^3\square$ Agree

   $^4\square$ Strongly agree

24. **When I left the hospital, I had a good understanding of the things I was responsible for in managing my health.**

   $^1\square$ Strongly disagree

   $^2\square$ Disagree

   $^3\square$ Agree

   $^4\square$ Strongly agree

25. **When I left the hospital, I clearly understood the purpose for taking each of my medications.**

   $^1\square$ Strongly disagree

   $^2\square$ Disagree

   $^3\square$ Agree

   $^4\square$ Strongly agree

   $^5\square$ I was not given any medication when I left the hospital

ABOUT YOU

There are only a few remaining items left.

26. **During this hospital stay, were you admitted to this hospital through the Emergency Room?**

   $^1\square$ Yes

   $^2\square$ No

27. **In general, how would you rate your overall health?**

   $^1\square$ Excellent

   $^2\square$ Very good

   $^3\square$ Good

   $^4\square$ Fair

   $^5\square$ Poor

28. **In general, how would you rate your overall mental or emotional health?**

   $^1\square$ Excellent

   $^2\square$ Very good

   $^3\square$ Good

   $^4\square$ Fair

   $^5\square$ Poor

29. **What is the highest grade or level of school that you have completed?**

   $^1\square$ 8th grade or less

   $^2\square$ Some high school, but did not graduate

   $^3\square$ High school graduate or GED

   $^4\square$ Some college or 2-year degree

   $^5\square$ 4-year college graduate

   $^6\square$ More than 4-year college degree

30. **Are you of Spanish, Hispanic or Latino origin or descent?**

   1 ☐ No, not Spanish/Hispanic/Latino
   2 ☐ Yes, Puerto Rican
   3 ☐ Yes, Mexican, Mexican American, Chicano
   4 ☐ Yes, Cuban
   5 ☐ Yes, other Spanish/Hispanic/Latino

31. **What is your race? Please choose one or more.**

   1 ☐ White
   2 ☐ Black or African American
   3 ☐ Asian
   4 ☐ Native Hawaiian or other Pacific Islander
   5 ☐ American Indian or Alaska Native

32. **What language do you <u>mainly</u> speak at home?**

   1 ☐ English
   2 ☐ Spanish
   3 ☐ Chinese
   4 ☐ Russian
   5 ☐ Vietnamese
   6 ☐ Portuguese
   9 ☐ Some other language (please print):

   _____

THANK YOU

Please return the completed survey in the postage-paid envelope.

[NAME OF SURVEY VENDOR OR SELF-ADMINISTERING HOSPITAL]

[RETURN ADDRESS OF SURVEY VENDOR OR SELF-ADMINISTERING HOSPITAL]

Sample Initial Cover Letter for the HCAHPS Survey

[HOSPITAL LETTERHEAD]

[SAMPLED PATIENT NAME]
[ADDRESS]
[CITY, STATE ZIP]

Dear [SAMPLED PATIENT NAME]:

Our records show that you were recently a patient at [NAME OF HOSPITAL] and discharged on [DATE OF DISCHARGE (mm/dd/yyyy)]. Because you had a recent hospital stay, we are asking for your help. This survey is part of an ongoing national effort to understand how patients view their hospital experience. Hospital results will be publicly reported and made available on the Internet at www.medicare.gov/hospitalcompare. These results will help consumers make important choices about their hospital care, and will help hospitals improve the care they provide.

Questions 1-25 in the enclosed survey are part of a national initiative sponsored by the United States Department of Health and Human Services to measure the quality of care in hospitals. Your participation is voluntary and will not affect your health benefits.

We hope that you will take the time to complete the survey. Your participation is greatly appreciated. After you have completed the survey, please return it in the prepaid envelope. Your answers may be shared with the hospital for purposes of quality improvement. [*OPTIONAL*: You may notice a number on the survey. This number is used to let us know if you returned your survey so we don't have to send you reminders.]

If you have any questions about the enclosed survey, please call the toll-free number 1-800-xxx-xxxx. Thank you for helping to improve health care for all consumers.

Sincerely,

[HOSPITAL ADMINISTRATOR]
[HOSPITAL NAME]

Note: The OMB Paperwork Reduction Act language must be included in the mailing. This language can be either on the front or back of the cover letter or questionnaire, but cannot be a separate mailing. The exact OMB Paperwork Reduction Act language is included in this appendix. Please refer to the Mail Only, and Mixed Mode sections, for specific letter guidelines.

Sample Follow-up Cover Letter for the HCAHPS Survey

[HOSPITAL LETTERHEAD]

[SAMPLED PATIENT NAME]
[ADDRESS]
[CITY, STATE ZIP]

Dear [SAMPLED PATIENT NAME]:

Our records show that you were recently a patient at [NAME OF HOSPITAL] and discharged on [DATE OF DISCHARGE (mm/dd/yyyy)]. Approximately three weeks ago we sent you a survey regarding your hospitalization. If you have already returned the survey to us, please accept our thanks and disregard this letter. However, if you have not yet completed the survey, please take a few minutes and complete it now.

Because you had a recent hospital stay, we are asking for your help. This survey is part of an ongoing national effort to understand how patients view their hospital experience. Hospital results will be publicly reported and made available on the Internet at www.medicare.gov/hospitalcompare. These results will help consumers make important choices about their hospital care, and will help hospitals improve the care they provide.

Questions 1-25 in the enclosed survey are part of a national initiative sponsored by the United States Department of Health and Human Services to measure the quality of care in hospitals. Your participation is voluntary and will not affect your health benefits. Please take a few minutes and complete the enclosed survey. After you have completed the survey, please return it in the prepaid envelope. Your answers may be shared with the hospital for purposes of quality improvement. [*OPTIONAL*: You may notice a number on the survey. This number is used to let us know if you returned your survey so we don't have to send you reminders.]

If you have any questions about the enclosed survey, please call the toll-free number 1-800-xxx-xxxx. Thank you again for helping to improve health care for all consumers.

Sincerely,

[HOSPITAL ADMINISTRATOR]
[HOSPITAL NAME]

Note: The OMB Paperwork Reduction Act language must be included in the mailing. This language can be either on the front or back of the cover letter or questionnaire, but cannot be a separate mailing. The exact OMB Paperwork Reduction Act language is included in this appendix. Please refer to the Mail Only, and Mixed Mode sections, for specific letter guidelines.

OMB Paperwork Reduction Act Language

The OMB Paperwork Reduction Act language must be included in the survey mailing. This language can be either on the front or back of the cover letter or questionnaire, but cannot be a separate mailing. The following is the language that must be used:

English Version

"According to the Paperwork Reduction Act of 1995, no persons are required to respond to a collection of information unless it displays a valid OMB control number. The valid OMB control number for this information collection is 0938-0981. The time required to complete this information collected is estimated to average 8 minutes for questions 1-25 on the survey, including the time to review instructions, search existing data resources, gather the data needed, and complete and review the information collection. If you have any comments concerning the accuracy of the time estimate(s) or suggestions for improving this form, please write to: Centers for Medicare & Medicaid Services, 7500 Security Boulevard, C1-25-05, Baltimore, MD 21244-1850."

Glossary

Acetabulum: The cup-shaped socket located on the side of the pelvis that makes up half of the hip joint. The head of the femur fits into the acetabulum.

Activities of Daily Living (ADLs): Daily personal habits such as toileting, bathing, dressing, showering, grooming, and eating; occupational therapists address difficulties patients have with these tasks after surgery.

Arthroplasty: *Arthro* means joint, *plasty* means to mold. Joint replacement is also called joint arthroplasty.

Assistive device: A walker, a pair of crutches, a cane, a wheelchair, a knee scooter; any device that aids in walking or moving; physical therapists identify the most appropriate devices and teach patients how to use them.

Axillary nerve: A nerve extending into the armpit that supplies several shoulder muscles, including the deltoids and one of the rotator cuff muscles as well as the triceps. Improper use of crutches can cause dysfunction of the axillary nerve.

Biceps: A two-part muscle on the front of the upper arm that bends or flexes the elbow.

Blood clot, also known as a **Deep Vein Thrombosis (DVT):** The platelets in our blood cause normal clotting, but if the flow of blood in a deep vein in the muscle tissue of the legs is compromised due to surgery or lack of movement, a larger abnormal clot can develop. If the clot travels to the lungs and blocks the flow of blood there, it is called a pulmonary embolism (PE), which can be fatal. Any surgery to the legs puts a patient at risk for blood clots. Long periods of inactivity, such as sitting on an airplane, also increase the risk. Blood-thinning medication is one tool used to preempt a blood clot. Other tools are ankle pumps, early walking, and compression pumps.

Breakthrough pain: Pain that occurs between normal doses of pain medication.

Cervical spine: The seven vertebrae in the neck, labeled C1 through C7.

Clavicle: The collarbone, located between the ribcage (sternum) and the shoulder blade (scapula); links the arm to the trunk of the body.

Evaluation: A patient's first visit with a physical or occupational therapist. This visit lasts longer because the therapist interviews the patient about the home, mobility constraints prior to surgery, the patient's goals, and equipment needs. Subsequent sessions are called Treatments. A doctor's order for therapy usually states "Eval and Treat."

Femoral head: The round ball at the top of the femur. It is removed in a total hip replacement.

Femur: The thigh bone. The longest and strongest bone in the body, it connects the hip to the knee.

Fibula: The outer bone in the lower leg, its low end forms part of the ankle joint.

Glenoid cavity: Also called the glenoid fossa. The receptacle of the humeral head, it's the saucer-shaped surface on the scapula that makes up half of the shoulder joint.

Humerus: The upper arm bone.

Humeral head: The round top of the upper arm bone. It fits into the glenoid cavity to form the shoulder joint, also known as the glenohumeral joint.

Goniometer: A handheld device resembling a protractor, used by physical therapists to measure the range of motion in a joint. Each joint has a normal range of motion, which is decreased after surgery. The tool allows for therapists to measure changes in movement objectively.

Hamstrings: The muscles responsible for bending the knee, also called knee flexion. They originate at the "sit" bones and back of the thigh and insert below the knee on the shinbone (tibia) and the outer leg bone (fibula). They bend the knee when they contract.

Hematoma: A pooling of blood that has leaked out of the capillaries and into the tissues, creating a hard, rubbery mass.

Hip abductors: The muscles on the buttocks and outside of the upper thigh that lift the leg out to the side, a movement called hip abduction. Usually weak after hip surgery and in the elderly population, these muscles are essential to good balance.

Hip extension: The movement of the thigh backward from a standing position, or upward when lying on the stomach. Muscles used are the gluts and the hamstrings.

Hip flexion: The movement of the thigh forward, as in a kicking motion, or lifting the knee up toward the chest. Hip flexion also occurs in bending forward from a standing position. Muscles used are called hip flexors.

Huddle: A morning meeting, or impromptu one, of clinicians from different disciplines to discuss the status of patients before they are seen that day, to bring everyone who is seeing each patient up to date.

Hypoxemia: The state of having insufficient oxygen in the arterial blood. Hypoxia, also a common term, refers to insufficient oxygen in the tissues. Hypoxemia can lead to hypoxia.

Knee extension: The movement of straightening the knee from a bent position. Can also refer to the knee in a static, straight position. Full knee extension is 0 degrees, as measured with a goniometer. Hyperextension is the state of an overstraightened knee.

Knee flexion: The movement of bending the knee from a straight position. Can also refer to the knee in a static, bent position. Full knee flexion is normally about 135 degrees, as measured with a goniometer.

Knee walker: An assistive device resembling a scooter, with two wheels in front and two in back, and a platform for one leg, often used by patients after an ankle replacement.

Latissimus dorsi: A large, broad muscle on each side of the back, it pulls the arm inward; it is active during crutch use.

Lumbar spine: The vertebrae of the low back, below the thoracic spine and above the sacrum, labeled L1 through L5.

Non-weight bearing (NWB): No weight may be placed on the limb that is non-weight bearing. An ankle patient who is NWB will need to use a walker, crutches, a knee scooter, or wheelchair. A shoulder patient who is NWB may not push off from or down on a surface with the affected arm or hand.

Orthopedics, aka **Orthopaedics:** *Ortho* means straight, *pedic* means foot; a branch of medicine concerned with the correction or prevention of deformities, disorders, or injuries of the musculoskeletal system, especially the extremities and the spine, and associated structures, as muscles and ligaments.

Patella: The kneecap.

Prehabilitation: Physical therapy provided before surgery and specifically tailored to prepare a patient; may consist of education and training with an assistive device.

Quadriceps: The muscles responsible for straightening the knee and the most essential to walking. They originate at the top of the thigh, and insert on the bony prominence below the kneecap. They straighten the knee when they contract.

Reciprocal gait: The normal human walking pattern, in which one leg advances along with the opposite arm. Physical therapy after surgery aims to restore this walking pattern.

Sacrum: The wedge-shaped base of the spinal column, it is below the lumbar spine and contains two vertebrae, S1 and S2.

Scapula: The shoulder blade. It contains the glenoid cavity.

Shoulder external rotation: A prohibited movement after total shoulder surgery, consisting of moving the hands out to the sides and away from the body from a starting position of bent elbows that hug the body; another version is a pitcher's stance just before throwing the ball.

Shoulder flexion: The movement of lifting the arm straight up in front of the body when standing, or lifting the arm in the air when lying down. Active lifting of the arm is a prohibited movement after total shoulder surgery, although passive lifting (having it lifted by the other arm or another person, without using your own muscles) is sometimes permitted.

Step-through pattern of walking: The normal, lower-body walking pattern, in which one leg advances, and the other leg advances past it.

Step-to pattern of walking: A compensatory pattern used after leg surgery in which the surgical leg advances, and the strong leg advances just far enough to meet it. This is the early walking pattern for post-op knee and hip patients.

Sternum: The breastbone, to which one end of the clavicle, or collarbone, attaches.

Talus: The uppermost bone of the foot, above the heel, that forms the ankle joint, together with the tibia and the fibula.

Thoracic spine: The middle section of the vertebral column, between the cervical and lumbar spine, labeled T1 through T12. All but the lowest two ribs connect to the thoracic spine, adding to its stability.

Tibia: The shinbone. It is the weight-bearing bone in the lower leg. Its upper surface is part of the knee joint and its lower surface is part of the ankle joint.

Triceps: A two-part muscle on the back surface of the humerus that straightens the elbow.

Vasovagal response or **syncope:** The most common type of fainting, sometimes preceded by paleness, clamminess, nausea and vomiting, symptoms that are brought on by a sudden decrease in blood pressure and heart rate that results in reduced blood flow to the brain. Not usually dangerous unless the patient falls, but orthopedic patients may need IV fluids after a vasovagal episode. The patient may also be placed in a position called Trendelenburg; lying flat on the back with the foot of the bed elevated, to promote blood flow to the brain.

Weight bearing as tolerated (WBAT): The status of most patients after knee and hip replacement, allowing patients to put as much weight as they can tolerate on the surgical leg when walking. Most patients still need an assistive device, such as a walker, crutches, or cane in the initial stages after surgery, for comfort, safety, and balance.

Endnotes

Introduction: What You Know Can Only Help You

1   www.OrthoColorado.org. The hospital is owned in part by Centura Health and in part by physicians, primarily members of Panorama Orthopedics in Golden, Colorado.

2   www.cms.gov/medicare/quality-initiatives-patient-assessment-instruments/ hospitalqualityinits/downloads/hospitalhcahpsfactsheet201007.pdf.
    Other articles on this topic: Jennifer White, "Improving Satisfaction after Primary Total Knee Arthroplasty Using Nurse Practitioner-Driver Preoperative Education," (2015) Doctoral Theses. Paper 13. and Mary Rechtoris, "7 Pillars for Success with Bundled Payments: Orthopedics and Beyond," *Becker's Spine Review*, November 8, 2016.

3   A payment plan called *bundling* was initiated in April 2016 for knee and hip replacements covered by Medicare. One reimbursement model stipulates that all expenses incurred in the first ninety days of the patient's care episode—including rehabilitation costs and readmission to the hospital—must be covered by the bundle.
    An orthopedic perspective on bundling can be found at www.aaos.org/ News/DailyEdition2016/Friday/013/?ssopc=1.

4   All of these surgeries are on the rise. Knees are the most commonly replaced joints, numbering more than 700,000 per year. Hips exceed 300,000. Shoulders add up to about 53,000. Ankle replacements are newer and number about 4,000. Spinal fusion surgeries number more than 413,000. Sources include www.cdc.gov/nchs/nhds, the Agency for Healthcare Research and Quality, orthoinfo.aaos.org, Orthopedixmd.com, and a study by S.S. Rajaee, et al., "Spinal Fusion in the United States: Analysis of Trends from 1998 to 2008," *Spine* (37 (1) (January 1, 2012): 67–76. According to an article by S. Kurtz, et al., "Projections of Primary and Revision Hip and Knee Arthroplasty in

the United States from 2005 to 2030," *Journal of Bone & Joint Surgery* 89 (4) (April 2007): 780–5, "By 2030, the demand for primary total hip arthroplasties is estimated to grow by 174% to 572,000. The demand for primary total knee arthroplasties is projected to grow by 673% to 3.48 million procedures."

5 At the Hospital for Special Surgery: health.usnews.com/best-hospitals/rankings/orthopedics?page=3.

6 A detailed description of the study, which was also presented at a 2016 meeting of the American Physical Therapy Association, is available at www.hss.edu/newsroom_hss-study-finds-patient-sessions-prepare-for-hip-and-knee-replacement.asp.

7 Another study about the value of preoperative patient education that is not mentioned in the text: Ioannis Papanastassiou, et al., "Effects of Preoperative Education on Spinal Surgery Patients," *International Journal of Spine Surgery* 5(4) (2011): 120–124. The authors write, "Of the participants in the pre-care class, 96% were satisfied with their pain management versus 83% in the control group. There was also a trend for better overall satisfaction in the pre-care class group."

Chapter 1: Choosing Your Surgeon

8 According to Wesley H. Bronson, et al., in "Ethics of Provider Risk Factor Modification in Total Joint Arthroplasty," *Journal of Bone & Joint Surgery* 97 (19) (October 7, 2015): 1635–1639, "Volume and experience are known to be predictive of better outcomes. Should all surgeons, regardless of volume or experience be allowed to perform joint replacements? Should all hospitals be permitted to offer hip and knee replacements to their patients?"

Chapter 2: Getting Ready for Surgery

9 Much has been written and videotaped about Dr. House's incorrect walking pattern. Here is a link to a short video: www.youtube.com/watch?v=lC6y7uMrNu0.

10 A paper was presented at a 2016 meeting of the American Academy of Orthopaedic Surgeons, by Matthew S. Austin, MD, "Formal Physical Therapy after Primary Total Hip Arthroplasty May Not Be Necessary."

Also see a blog post by Robert H. Shmerling of Harvard Health Publications: www.health.harvard.edu/blog/physical-therapy-hip-replacement-can-rehab-happen-home-201605119563.

11 Evan L. Flatow, MD, and Alicia K. Harrison, MD, "A History of Reverse Total Shoulder Arthroplasty," *Clinical Orthopaedics and Related Research* 469 (9) (September 2001): 2432–2439.

   Another citation about the FDA approval in 2004 can be found at www. hopkinsmedicine.org/orthopaedic-surgery/specialty-areas/shoulder/treat-ments-procedures/reverse-prosthesis.html.

12 To see if your state allows you to see a physical therapist without a doctor's prescription, go to https://www.apta.org/uploadedFiles/APTAorg/Advocacy/State/Issues/Direct_Access/DirectAccessbyState.pdf.

Chapter 3: You Can't Go Home Alone

13 The story has two parts, appearing in Medscape. The first, "When a Knee Replacement Specialist Needs His Own Knee," appeared September 7, 2016. The second, "Part 2: When a Knee Replacement Specialist Needs His Own Knee," appeared October 5, 2016.

   His knee was replaced on an outpatient basis, and he recuperated at his surgeon's home. His story makes for informative reading for prospective knee-replacement patients.

Chapter 4: Know Your Lines

14 For a favorable look at the machine, go to www.mykneeguide.com/the-hospi-tal/cpm-machine, watch the video, and read the blog by Brian Hatten, MD, revised 5/31/2016. One error in the video: you will not achieve 120 degrees of knee flexion in the machine. Once you reach 90 degrees (or less), your hip will become too uncomfortable to stay in the machine.

   Most scientific studies of CPMs show that they provide no benefit imme-diately after recovery and that their use may result in longer-lasting postop-erative swelling. For a quick take, read the abstract of "To use or not to use continuous passive motion post-total knee arthroplasty presenting functional assessment results in early recovery," by R.N. Manier, et al., *Journal of Arthro-plasty* 27 (2) (February 2012): 193–200.

Chapter 5: Who's Who in the Hospital

15 Taro Okamoto, et al., "Day-of-Surgery Mobilization Reduces the Length of Stay After Elective Hip Arthroplasty," *Journal of Arthroplasty* (10) (October 31, 2016): 2227–2230.

16 For a history of the hospitalist movement, go to en.wikipedia.org/wiki/ Hospital_medicine.

Chapter 6: Personal Demons

17 Nicholas Giori, MD, and Alex Harris, MD, presented their findings at the American Academy of Orthopaedic Surgeons (AAOS) 2011 Annual Meeting: Abstract P040. Presented February 15, 2011. Details can be found in an article by Fran Lowry, "Alcohol Linked to Complications after Joint Surgery," in *Health News*, February 18, 2011.

18 For an explanation of alcohol's effects on the body, go to the site: alcoholrehab.com/alcoholism/problem-drinker-defined/ or to www.niaaa.nih.gov.

19 The CIWA scale is available at www.umem.org/files/uploads/1104212257_ CIWA-Ar.pdf.

20 H. Maradit-Kremers H, et al., "Social and Behavioral Factors in Total Knee and Hip Arthroplasty," *Journal of Arthroplasty* 30 (10) (October 2015): 1852–1854.

21 Jasvinder A. Singh, et al., "Current Tobacco Use is Associated with Higher Rates of Implant Revision and Deep Infection after Total Hip or Knee Arthroplasty: A Prospective Cohort Study," *BMC Med* 13 (2015): 283.

22 After determining your BMI at www.cdc.gov/healthyweight/assessing/bmi/ adult_bmi/english_bmi_calculator/bmi_calculator.html, follow the link to About BMI for Adults.

23 Hasham M. Alvi, MD, et al., "The Effect of BMI on 30-Day Outcomes Following Total Joint Arthroplasty," *Journal of Arthroplasty* 30 (7) (July 2015): 1113–1117.

24 Eric M. Wagner, MD, et al., "The Effect of Body Mass Index on Reoperation and Complications after Total Knee Arthroplasty," *Journal of Bone & Joint Surgery* 98 (24) (December 21, 2016): 2052–2060.

25 Afshin A. Anoushiravani, BSc, et al., "Assessing In-Hospital Outcomes and Resource Utilization after Primary Total Joint Arthroplasty among Underweight Patients," *Journal of Arthroplasty* 31 (7) (July 2016): 1407–1412.

26 For a definition of tolerance, dependency, and addiction, see www.webmd. com/pain-management/features/pain-medication-addiction#2.

27 Jenna Goesling, et al., "Trends and Predictors of Opioid Use after Total Knee and Total Hip Arthroplasty," *Pain* 157 (6) (June 2016):1259–1265.

Chapter 7: Coping with Pain

28 For additional reading on this topic, see Amish J. Dave, MD, et al., "Is There an Association Between Whole-body Pain with Osteoarthritis-related Knee Pain, Pain Catastrophizing, and Mental Health?" *Clinical Orthopedics Related Research* 473 (2015): 3894–3902.

29 For an interesting article on pain, go to www.webmd.com/pain-management/features/pain-scale. Then click on images to see the visual analog scale.

30 The removal of pain as the fifth vital sign occurred in 6/2016. See www.painnewsnetwork.org/stories/2016/6/16/ama-drops-pain-as-vital-sign. This doesn't mean pain is ignored or considered insignificant. But the AMA action differentiates pain from the four other vital signs, all of which can be objectively measured.

31 www.cdc.gov/drugoverdose/data/overdose.html.

32 www.nytimes.com/2014/02/03/movies/philip-seymour-hoffman-actor-dies-at-46.html?_r=0.

33 www.cdc.gov/drugoverdose/data/heroin.html.

34 www.painnewsnetwork.org/stories/2016/2/18/guidelines-for-post-surgical-pain-discourage-use.

35 For a discussion of the merits of the newer Lyrica versus the older Neurontin (or pregabalin versus gabapentin) in total joint surgery, go to www.newhealthguide.org/Lyrica-vs-Gabapentin.html.

Chapter 8: Rehab Starts Now

36 The type and amount of therapy ordered varies significantly from state to state, hospital to hospital, and surgeon to surgeon. The information in this chapter gives you a general idea of what to expect, but your experience may differ. My advice is to advocate for what you think you need.

Chapter 9: The ABCs of Hospital Culture

37 For more information on the history of HCAHPS, go to www.hcahpsonline.org/files/HCAHPS%20Fact%20Sheet,%20revised1,%203-31-09.pdf.

38 Three articles of interest include, Alexandra Robbins, "The Problem with Satisfied Patients," *The Atlantic,* April 17, 2015; Rick Evans, "There's a Difference between Happy and Satisfied Patients," *Policy,* August 6, 2015; and Heather Punke, "Are Patient Satisfaction Surveys Doing More Harm than Good," *Becker's Infection Control and Clinical Quality,* June 9, 2015.

39 Health.usnews.com/health-news/patient-advice/articles/2015/10/15/
    the-patient-wish-list.

    Johns Hopkins Medicine has a chief patient experience officer. It is also
    home to the Armstrong Institute, which is headed by Peter Pronovost, a lead-
    ing authority on patient safety.

Chapter 10: Homeward Bound

40 K. J. DiSilvestro, et al., "When Can I Drive after Orthopaedic Surgery? A
    Systematic Review," *Clinical Orthopaedics and Related Research* 474 (12)
    (December 2016): 2557–2570.

41 www.aahks.org/care-for-hips-and-knees/do-i-need-a-joint-replacement/
    total-hip-replacement/.

    AAHKS stands for the American Association of Hip and Knee Surgeons.

42 C.C. Johnson, et al., "Return to Sports after Shoulder Arthroplasty," *World
    Journal of Orthopedics* 7 (9) (September 18, 2016): 519–526.

43 E.C. McCarty, et al., "Sport Participation after Shoulder Replacement Sur-
    gery," *American Journal of Sports Medicine* 36 (8) (August 2008): 1577–1581.

44 www.columbiaortho.org/sites/default/files/u3/Sports_Total_Shoulder_Jobin.

45 R.W. Molinari, et al., "Return to Play in Athletes Receiving Cervical Surgery:
    A Systematic Review," *Global Spine Journal* 6 (1) (February 2016): 89–96.

    D.G. Kang, et al., "Return to Play after Cervical Disc Surgery," *Clinical
    Sports Medicine* 35 (4) (October 2016): 529–543.

46 M.G. Burnett and V.K. Sonntag, "Return to Contact Sports after Spinal Sur-
    gery," *Neurosurgery Focus*, 21 (4) (2006): E-5.

47 G.D. Shifflett, et al., "Return to Golf After Lumbar Fusion," *Sports Health*,
    November 22, 2016.

48 F.D. Naal, et al., "Habitual Physical Activity and Sports Participation after
    Total Ankle Arthroplasty," *American Journal of Sports Medicine* 37 (1) (Janu-
    ary 2009): 95–102.

Index

Acknowledgments

Jared Foran, MD, is a force of nature, someone who seemingly punctuates everything he does with exclamation marks. Just two years after his arrival at OrthoColorado and the neighboring St. Anthony Hospital in Lakewood, Colorado, he became the director of the joint replacement programs at both. He also serves as the joint replacement section editor for the American Academy of Orthopaedic Surgeons' excellent website (ortho-info.org). Dr. Foran agreed generously and without hesitation to help with this book, writing the foreword, answering many questions, critiquing the manuscript (with exclamation marks), and referring me to other experts. A prolific surgeon, he never once said he was too busy to help. I'm extremely grateful for his support.

I also want to thank William Peace, MD, for sharing his expertise about hip replacement; David Schneider, MD, for shoulder replacement; Mark Conklin, MD, for total ankle replacement, and Lonnie Loutzenhiser, MD, for spine fusion surgery. All of these orthopedic surgeons gave thoughtful answers to my pages of questions. Thanks also to the Hospital for Special Surgery professionals in New York who answered my questions about physical therapy. HSS also has an excellent patient education website.

Thanks to my son, Travis Tucker, for taking the photographs in Chapter 2, and to my good friend Nancy Orr, who modeled for them. Trav and his brother Cam also cheered me on through this process and assisted with technical difficulties, usually telling me to just google it.

Thanks to my readers, who gave generously of their time: Parry Burnap, Susan Grosso, RN, my brother Rod Kaufmann, Sibylle Keller, my sister-in-law Barbara Philipps, and Tracy Poepping, NP; and a special thanks to Nora Sullivan, PT, OCS; Nikki Sobotka, DPT; and writer Lauren Ward

Larsen, all of whom honed in on details and concepts with exceptional insight and thoughtfulness.

Shari Caudron, MFA, thank you for helping me shape this idea and bring it to fruition.

Thanks to my agent, Steve Harris, and to Skyhorse editorial director Joseph Craig for believing in this project. Michael Campbell at Skyhorse also deserves credit for jumping in at the end of this project and putting it to bed.

Thanks also to my brother C. B. Kaufmann, my sister-in-law Patty Kaufmann, my sister-in-law Margaret Tucker, and to the many friends who supported me in various ways, including writers Francine Mathews, Jennifer Parmelee, and Sherrye Henry, MFA; Meg Leonard and Michael Leonard, MD; Francie Fowler, Therese Lincoln, Sarah Lamm White, PsyD, Tanya Hyland, PT, Sara Calaway White, Elizabeth Wald, Idske Hiemstra, and Anne Murdaugh.

About the Author

Elizabeth Kaufmann is a writer and physical therapist who grew up in Munich, Germany, and Connecticut. She received her undergraduate degree from Yale and worked as a staff editor for *Audubon* and *Outside* magazines before launching a freelance writing career. Her work appeared in those magazines as well as the *New York Times, Shape, Self,* and others. She covered the 1987 Snowbird Everest Expedition for the *Chicago Tribune*, penning stories in her tent at the eighteen-thousand-foot base camp.

Pursuing a deeper interest in health and fitness, she wrote a childbirth book, *Vaginal Birth after Cesarean/The Smart Woman's Guide to VBAC*, then earned a master's degree in physical therapy from Northwestern Medical School. She worked as a physical therapist in orthopedics and trauma and also the AIDS ward at Cook County Hospital in Chicago before moving with her family to Evergreen, Colorado, in 2001. She worked for Mt. Evans Home Health Care and Hospice in Evergreen, then for St. Anthony Central Hospital in Denver, specializing in orthopedics and trauma; she transferred to OrthoColorado Hospital in Lakewood when it opened in 2010. She and her husband, writer Ernest Tucker, have two sons, the aforementioned Trav and Cam. She enjoys downhill skiing, tennis, hiking, biking, yoga, horseback riding, and photography.